Life and Death in Rikers Island

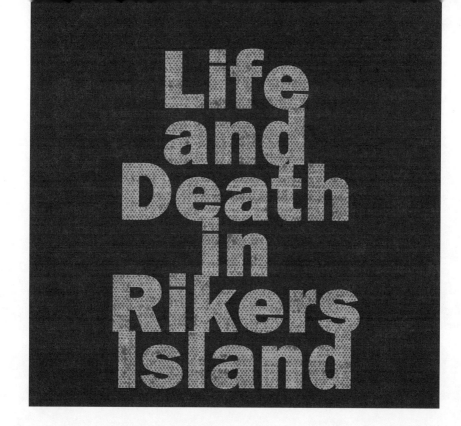

Life and Death in Rikers Island

Homer Venters

Former Chief Medical Officer of NYC Jails

JOHNS HOPKINS UNIVERSITY PRESS

Baltimore

To Susan. You know what you did.

© 2019 Johns Hopkins University Press
All rights reserved. Published 2019
Printed in the United States of America on acid-free paper
9 8 7 6 5 4 3 2 1

Johns Hopkins University Press
2715 North Charles Street
Baltimore, Maryland 21218-4363
www.press.jhu.edu

Library of Congress Cataloging-in-Publication Data

Names: Venters, Homer, 1967– author.
Title: Life and death in Rikers Island / Homer Venters.
Description: Baltimore : Johns Hopkins University Press, 2019. | Includes
    bibliographical references and index.
Identifiers: LCCN 2018023724 | ISBN 9781421427355 (pbk. : alk. paper) |
    ISBN 9781421427362 (electronic) | ISBN 1421427354 (pbk. : alk. paper) |
    ISBN 1421427362 (electronic)
Subjects: | MESH: New York (N.Y.). Department of Correction. | Prisons |
    Delivery of Health Care | Prisoners | Health Status | Health Risk Behaviors |
    Human Rights Abuses | New York City
Classification: LCC RA448.N5 | NLM WA 300 AN7 | DDC 362.109747/1—dc23
LC record available at https://lccn.loc.gov/2018023724

A catalog record for this book is available from the British Library.

*Special discounts are available for bulk purchases of this book. For more information, please
contact Special Sales at 410-516-6936 or specialsales@press.jhu.edu.*

Johns Hopkins University Press uses environmentally friendly book materials,
including recycled text paper that is composed of at least 30 percent post-consumer
waste, whenever possible.

Contents

Contents

Acknowledgments

THERE ARE MANY PEOPLE who have opened my eyes to the health risks of jail. I've benefited from working with a team of mission-driven people who have improved the lives of many thousands of patients in our time together. I've mentioned some of the key members and programs of this team throughout this book, but every member of correctional health services deserves tremendous respect for the work they do. I will discuss the nursing, medical, data, and mental health services often throughout, but a few other programs deserve acknowledgment for advancing our mission to document and reduce the health risks of jail. Our IT team in the jail correctional health service, led by Rick Stazesky, enabled us to simultaneously deliver care and capture data to detect abuse. Without this team, we could not have conducted most of our reports on health outcomes. Tom Hayden and his pharmacy team probably have the most objective and total view of the jails because of their ability to work in clinics; to monitor small, remote pharmacy windows; and even to bring medications to housing areas.

There have been several outside partners in our work who left before I did. The first is the former Department of Correction (DOC) deputy commissioner Erik Berliner. Erik was my counterpart at DOC, and we more or less came up the ranks together. His unit of DOC, called Health Affairs, existed to coordinate with us in the health unit on the many issues we shared, such as patient production, clinic productivity, and staff squabbles. I sometimes describe Health Affairs as the curtain to our tennis ball, there to soak up our kinetic energy without disturbing the security leaders. When he left the DOC about two years ago, we lost a true partner to our health service. He wasn't able to effect change in DOC on some critical issues, but he and I shared a strategic plan on how to cooperate most of the time and work around each other when we couldn't find common ground. He deserves as much credit as anyone for design of the clinical alternatives to solitary confinement units that would allow us to remove seriously mentally ill patients from solitary. Even when our agencies were headed for conflict, we had an open line of communication that helped limit harm to patients and staff.

Another partner I need to acknowledge is Cathy Potler, who was executive director of our oversight board before she passed away. Cathy was the most zealous and unapologetic advocate for our patients whom I encountered during my time in the jails. She worked tirelessly to steer her oversight body toward a more active role in holding DOC and us in correctional health accountable for compliance with basic laws and rules. During my time as medical director and assistant commissioner, she and I worked very closely to document abuse of patients and strategized how best to proceed on almost every case we encountered. Her requests for information and accountability by DOC would irritate and then anger an entire agency. Ultimately, DOC began to spend considerable amounts of time complaining to city hall about Cathy and her requests for basic data and explanations of practices. Cathy had already developed an entire career in promoting human rights, and with the staunch support of her son and husband, she seemed unaffected by the pushback from DOC and city hall. Dr. Bobby Cohen was (and remains) a member of the oversight board that Cathy led. Bobby has also been a longtime mentor to me, and for several years Bobby's and Cathy's voices were quite alone, as a chorus of other NYC officials would proclaim that things were fine or improving in the jails. Had those same officials spent less time trying to marginalize Cathy, Bobby, and others raising the alert, Rikers might be closed today. About a year before her death, I brought Cathy a bottle of wine to celebrate some hopeful test results about her cancer. I was so struck that in the face of life-threatening illness she wouldn't give one inch to the system that worked so hard to marginalize her and harm the incarcerated.

There are a host of others whom I will acknowledge in the pages that follow. I've been very fortunate to have great bosses, each of whom helped me to advance this mission at critical times and protect me at others. Maria Gbur recruited me to come be her deputy right out of fellowship, and she was a fierce and feared advocate for patient care. Louise Cohen, Amanda Parsons, and Sonia Angell were my bosses as deputy commissioners at the NYC Department of Health and Mental Hygiene, and they all gave me great support in establishing the human rights framework to correctional health. They also taught me a tremendous amount about their areas of expertise, including primary care, information technology, and chronic disease management. My recent boss at NYC Health + Hospitals, Patsy Yang, has been a tireless advocate for increasing the funding and scope of services of correctional health, and she will be a zealous guardian of our resources in coming years. I've been able to manage the tougher stretches of this work thanks to some close and insightful confidants, including Ross MacDonald and Cecilia Flaherty, our chief of medicine and director of programs, respectively.

Our mission has also benefited from the counsel (and criticism) of groups outside correctional health, namely, a crew of progressive city council members whom I will mention later in the book, advocates like Jennifer Parrish at Urban Justice, and prisoners' rights lawyers such as Dale Wilker, Sarah Kerr, John Boston, Riley Evans, and Jonathan Chassan.

My early thoughts about the health risks of jail were really influenced by quarterly meetings we set up called the Human Rights Collective. We would invite academics, professionals, advocates, and people with lived experience of incarceration to discuss difficult issues like solitary confinement, sexual violence, or racial disparities in care and punishment. These partners would teach us about some of the grim realities at play in the jails that had a major impact on the health of our patients and our ability to deliver ethical care. At one of these meetings, we started to dig into the problem of tracking and reporting abuse much more comprehensively, and a longtime research mentor, Dr. Ernie Drucker, commented that jail exposure was like being dipped in acid and then being put back in the community. This idea, along with the many partners we met with from outside our health service, helped me to appreciate the deadly and long-lasting health risks of jail.

Much of this book was written in the evenings, as I sat in our boys' room while they and their sister resisted going to sleep. Anthony and Drae turned 5 and Georgia 7 during the writing of this book, and they deserve a lot of credit for their patience with me. Plenty of others in my family and neighborhood have made this work and this book possible. I started seeing patients in the jails late Friday nights who had been hurt in DOC uses of force about the same time we moved to our current neighborhood. Our neighbors, Rob and Caroline and Ben and Andrea, had beers on hand after many of those nights, and I really appreciated their kindness when I came home wild-eyed, wound up, or upset. My wife, Susan, has been my main sounding board for every issue at work and has given me many smart ideas to improve this book.

Like every book written by a doctor, the final acknowledgment goes to my patients. This book delves into some ugly and horrible harms that the jail system visited on them. My goal in relating their stories, as well as the data we've analyzed, is to show the role of the jail system in their trauma, injuries, and deaths. Some of the people profiled in this book posed very difficult management challenges for security staff. Others simply didn't understand the rules of the jails or had the misfortune to need health care. But for every one of them, their safety and well-being were the responsibility of the jail system. The systemic failures of the jail system became their personal health risks. My goal is to provide an honest assessment of exactly how jail creates these health risks and to reveal the true costs of incarceration and the benefit of alternative strategies.

Life and Death in Rikers Island

Introduction

NCARCERATION HARMS HEALTH. In the United States, we have become the world's most voracious jailers, without truly understanding how the places where we send people increase their risk for death and serious injury. Despite sporadic news stories about horrible deaths, beatings, or sexual assaults in jail, we blame the incarcerated for whatever might happen to them behind bars. These are the bad guys, just getting what they deserve, or so we think.

While incarceration brings intrinsic health risks, we shouldn't ignore the preexisting health problems of the incarcerated. In fact, the health risks of incarceration are often connected to the very profiles of people whom we seem hungry to lock up. People of color, people living in poverty, people with mental health and substance use problems—these are the people whom we've steered toward jails and prisons over the past 30 years, and we've designed jails and prisons to expose them to major health risks. These personal characteristics play a large role in the likelihood of death, injury, or sickness while locked up. The health risks that jail or prison brings to bear on the incarcerated—such as violence, blocked access to care, and solitary confinement—disproportionately impact those with behavioral health problems and people of color.

In directing the health service in the New York City jail system, I've come to believe that accounting for the health risks of the jail system is one of our core responsibilities. Much can and should be done to improve basic health services in jail, and the team I've had the honor to work with in the NYC jails has made great strides in improving medical and mental health

1

care for our patients. But our responsibility to them doesn't end when they receive their medication or have an illness treated. Correctional health services like ours see every day how jail harms our patients, and we also possess the resources and skills to group together many health outcomes like injuries or sexual assaults and identify trends and risk factors. We owe our patients and the community at large a more honest assessment of what happens in jail to impact health during and after incarceration. This perspective is new and continues to be met with suspicion years after we've started to discuss it, largely because any discussion of health in jail is usually subordinated to the interests of the security authority and other governmental risk managers. This role is all the more critical because we work in settings that are designed and operated to keep the truth hidden. Detainees are beaten and threatened to prevent them from telling the truth about how they are injured, health staff are pressured to lie or omit details in their own documentation, and families experience systematic abuse and humiliation during the visitation process. Promoting a systematic approach to correctional health rarely occurs in the United States, largely because these systems are subordinate to the interests of security forces and their political supporters. But our lesson in the NYC jail system is that progress can be made in finding and telling the truth about the health risks of jail. To do so requires the tools of human rights, medicine, and epidemiology, and this can place the correctional health service at odds with the security service, other government officials, and even more traditional public health and medical institutions.

There are many health risks of jail, and I present some of them here through the stories of real people who were harmed during their time in the NYC jail system. For some of the health risks, like death and sexual assault, there is quite a bit of data outside our jail system that helps us to understand these stories. For other areas, like solitary confinement, injuries, and human rights, not much has been reported for US jails other than Rikers. This lack of data or analysis is not a surprise, since jails are paramilitary settings, where the group that has the health data is usually under the control of the security service. The stories of individual patients in Rikers are all taken from public accounts in newspapers, magazines, court filings, or various oversight reports. Many of the people mentioned in this book I knew personally.[1] I saw some of these patients routinely, others as they lay battered and bleeding after horrible violence. Some of them were defiant and outraged at what had happened to them, while others were reduced to tears. Many were stoic or "checked out." They knew the rules of the jail far better than I did and focused on their own survival. Some patients I first saw as they lay on an autopsy table, with telltale signs of abuse or neglect: bellies full of blood, broken bones, or organs overcome with infection. Often, when first responding to these circumstances, I would find myself in housing areas of the jails, with patients, correction officers, and medical staff all giving me their account of what had happened. As time passed working at Rikers, I became less certain of the categorical truth of one group or another. Instead, I came to appreciate that we often could not be sure of the truth and that many parts of the jail system were actually designed to keep the truth from our eyes.

LET'S BEGIN WITH THE STORY of J. W. Gamble. Mr. Gamble was incarcerated in Texas in 1973 and became injured that year when a 600-pound bale of hay fell onto him while he was working as an inmate. He received sporadic and inadequate medical care, and when he refused to return to his work detail because of untreated back injury and pain, he received disciplinary infractions from security staff and was placed in solitary confinement. He submitted a handwritten lawsuit against the Texas Department of Corrections, alleging that his constitutional rights had been violated, and, after several dismissals, his case ultimately went to the US Supreme Court. In 1976, the court ruled in his favor and established the principle that denial of medical care for the incarcerated constitutes deliberate indifference and meets the burden of cruel and unusual punishment, which is prohibited by the US Constitution's Eighth Amendment.[2] This case, *Estelle v. Gamble*, established the right to health care for prisoners in the United States, making them the only group with this constitutional guarantee.

In the 40 years since, we have dramatically expanded incarceration without addressing the many ways in which incarcerated people face new risks of injury, sickness, and death behind bars. The deaths, injuries, sickness, and trauma *caused* by incarceration are not part of our discussions about criminal justice because they are hidden. The money spent to respond to these failures, in lawsuits and health care after incarceration, is also generally hidden from public view. The legacy of *Estelle v. Gamble* is a national standard of care that, while improved from nothing, is still inadequate and often serves to hide the harms of incarceration, not reveal them. If we can become honest about the health risks of incarceration, then we can account for the full human and financial costs of going to jail and proceed to reduce these risks while also correcting the terrible American legacy of mass incarceration. Many of the cases included in this book have taken a path eerily similar to Mr. Gamble's, with a failure of care while incarcerated leading to a devastating health outcome and lawsuit against the detaining authority (see table A.1).

Before I started with correctional health services, two patients, Guido Newbrough and Scott Ortiz, pulled me into the intersection of health, human rights, and incarceration. Looking back, becoming involved in their cases helped to crystalize the path I've pursued. One of these patients died before I ever heard his name, while the other was awaiting sentencing when his lawyer reached out to me. Both of these cases left me motivated and angry, with the sense that incarceration is a space of common and profound abuse, neglect, and substandard care for patients.

Several years before joining the NYC correctional health service, I started my residency at Montefiore Medical Center in social internal medicine. Unbeknownst to me, a series of earlier medical directors at the NYC jail service were products of Montefiore, including Bert King, Bobby Cohen, and Steve Safyer. All three physicians would give me wise counsel when I finally followed in their footsteps. One of the skills we learned at Montefiore, documenting torture among people seeking asylum in the United States, would help me immeasurably a few years later when I started to look into abuse of patients in the NYC jail system.

As a social medicine resident at Montefiore, I often heard from formerly incarcerated patients how tough it was to access health care. The legal defense group Bronx Defenders was located practically across the street from our clinic in the South Bronx, so I set up a small project to have office hours in the Bronx Defenders offices. Once or twice a week, the social workers at Bronx Defenders would arrange for their clients to meet with me to discuss their health issues. One of the early and lasting lessons from these interactions was just how inaccessible our own clinic was for people coming out of jail.[3]

During my office hours at Bronx Defenders, one of the social workers, Jesse Lainer-Voss, asked for my help with the case of a client facing a long sentence for burglary. This client, Scott Ortiz, had several prior convictions for burglary, and the prosecutors were aiming to label him a predicate felon, meaning that his new burglary case could result in a 15-year sentence. Mr. Ortiz had HIV and advanced hepatitis C and was fairly incapacitated. I reviewed his case and testified at his sentencing hearing, making the point that his advanced liver failure was associated with a shortened life span. The judge decided to sentence Mr. Ortiz to 15 years as a predicate felon, which wasn't a shock. But when I received the judge's opinion, I struggled to believe what I was reading. The judge acknowledged that if he sentenced Mr. Ortiz to the regular sentence of two to four years for his burglary, he might not even survive that incarceration. But, he added, "given his weakened state, any assertion that the Defendant is a serious threat to the public as a burglar is really not credible. However, if released, he may well return to the life of a street addict, thereby endangering the public health through the exchange or sharing of dirty needles." During the trial, there had been no evidence or allegation of intravenous heroin use, and in fact, by all accounts, Mr. Ortiz had not used intravenous heroin for more than a decade. Reading how this judge was able to warp his supposed concern for public health into a justification for punishment was maddening, but it helped me focus on the bigotry that exists toward persons involved in both health and criminal justice systems. Unable to do much else, I wrote a paper with Mr. Ortiz's social work team on the judge's decision, which was published in the *Harm Reduction Journal*.[4] Documenting this misuse of public health as a pretext for incarceration was helpful for our team in processing the outcome, but for me, it also laid the groundwork for operationalizing a human rights approach; sometimes we can't fix the systemic problems that harm our patients, but we certainly can report how the "justice" system runs headlong into our mission to promote health.

A second patient would bring this message home a couple of years later, when I was working as a fellow to research health care in the Immigration and Customs Enforcement (ICE) network of detention centers.[5] During this work, I was contacted by Nina Bernstein, a journalist from the *New York Times*, who was working with the family of a man who had died in ICE detention. This man, Guido Newbrough, had become ill in a detention center in Virginia, and his increasing complaints of urinary incontinence, back pain, and lower extremity weakness were met with scorn and, eventually, a solitary confinement cell, where he died of blood infection.[6] Aside from the shocking abuse and neglect that he received from the security staff, his case introduced me to the very routine acts of humanity that the incarcerated show toward each other. As Mr. Newbrough's pain worsened over two weeks, the other detainees in his unit took turns making warm compresses for his back, and they ultimately took to banging on locked doors to get attention for him. Sometimes the only ray of hope in these cases is the compassion that people display toward each other in the face of neglect or abuse. In another ICE case I wrote about, a patient with AIDS was repeatedly denied basic medications to prevent opportunistic infection, and she became ill and died from one of these infections.[7] This patient was transgender and elicited scorn and neglect from both security and health staff in her detention facility. But as her infection worsened and she developed profuse vomiting, diarrhea, and hallucinations, it was the other detainees around her who staged a mass protest to trigger her transfer to the hospital, where she tragically died handcuffed to a bed.[8]

Health care is not a top priority in jail. That may sound obvious to those who look in from the outside, or those who actually go to jail or prison, but this truth is often countered by pointing to the many processes and resources dedicated to provision of health services. In the NYC correctional health service, we consider every "inmate" to be a "patient," partly because we do a rigorous medical and mental health intake for every person who arrives in jail, and partly because we want to keep focus on the independence of our mission. Unfortunately, health systems in jail and prison are usually designed and controlled by people who aren't health experts. In addition, the failures of the health systems behind bars are mostly hidden and, aside from when they result in death, rarely result in any calls for change. As a result, many of the health risks of jail are structural, arising from the basic design of the jail. For example, in 2013, the NYC jail system moved from a policy of allowing most patients to walk freely to the clinic (unescorted movement) to one of mostly needing escorts for movement. The idea was that violence would be reduced if a person going to a medical appointment or other activity outside their housing area were taken by a correctional officer "escort," who could take a few people to various destinations. What became quickly apparent was that there would never be enough of these escort officers to bring people to and from their basic activities in the jails, like healthcare encounters, meetings with lawyers, visits with families, recreation, and so on. This fundamental change cut deeply into patient production, meaning our ability to see patients. As a result, almost half of our appointments were missed at any given time. In the hardest-hit jails, we would give security staff list after list of the "must see" patients whom we feared might die without receiving care. Inevitably, as we pushed hard for a few weeks or months on mental health encounters, patient production would creep up, and medical or nursing or pharmacy production would plummet. Or we might make a brief improvement in a few types of patient production, and then a friendly deputy warden would be promoted, transferred, or fired, and we would fall back to half or fewer of our patients being produced. This type of change had a major effect on patient access to our health services, but as the leaders of the health service, we were never part of the discussion about whether or how to implement it, or involved in evaluating any evidence that it would actually decrease violence, which it did not.

No practice better exemplifies how the health mission is mangled by security priorities than solitary confinement. Solitary confinement is a practice that began in the modern age as a response to riots at a single prison, in Marion, Illinois, in 1983, and quickly became a common feature of prisons and jails across the United States. The only evidence to support this national policy change was the opinion of wardens and sheriffs that keeping people caged for 23 or 24 hours a day was safer for staff. Nothing stronger was ever presented in support of this strategy. When I began as assistant commissioner in 2011, the DOC asked us to agree to expansion of a solitary confinement unit for mentally ill prisoners. Even with my limited mental health background, this seemed like a horrible idea, and I put together a memo to my boss to argue that this unit should be closed rather than expanded. Almost all the senior health staff in correctional health, as well as some at Bellevue Hospital, signed onto this memo, but we were combatting the correctional opinion with our own contrary opinions. We were also stepping into a massive power imbalance, pitting our medical opinions about the welfare of our patients against the practices and cultural beliefs of the security service. We were able to hold off efforts to expand solitary for mentally ill patients and turn our attention to a larger-scale analysis of how solitary is actually associated with death and injury. After discussing with NYC health commissioner Tom Farley, we undertook the analysis presented later in this book, and we were able to join our data with the voices of many others against this practice. But who has demanded that the security leaders around the United States prove the utility, safety, or cost-effectiveness of solitary confinement? Until recently, nobody.

Over the past nine years, our efforts to document the health risks of jail have succeeded because of a core of bright, mission-driven staff, some with clinical skills and some with purely analytic skills. Their names are on the articles I cite in this book, and their efforts have carved out an important space for the notion that correctional health can improve on care while also documenting the health risks of incarceration. I can recall the first time one of our core researchers, Fatos Kaba, raised the issue of traumatic brain injury with me in 2009, when I was the deputy medical director. It seemed like an interesting but academic issue, but her persistence and my own experience with patients kept it alive as a research question until we could dedicate resources to it in 2011. Fatos's zeal for this topic would spawn important spin-offs for two other young researchers, Jasmine Graves and Cassandra Ramdath, who pushed our initial work into the realms of structural violence and neuroscience. Working with this team and benefiting from their zeal to help our patients has made these years incredibly fulfilling, when they could have been bleak. We have analyzed multiple health risks in jail, including injuries, sexual assault, solitary confinement, and even the racial disparities in our mental health service. When we began our efforts, most of what we did was partially hidden because of numerous objections to our efforts. As we gained support from our own agency, and as our data fell into the right hands, including the US Department of Justice (DOJ), we gathered steam. The DOJ's investigation into brutality by security staff was initiated by US Attorney Preet Bharara and ushered in a wave of scrutiny by others, including the press, state investigators, and the New York City Council. Without this investigation, many of the terrifying personal stories and systemic analyses included in this book would have remained in the shadows. Along the way, every one of my bosses has helped at a critical time, including Health Commissioners Farley and Bassett. This work allowed a highly skilled team of health providers to analyze data in our electronic medical record to improve the quality of care and also document the health risks of incarceration. This mission has also developed leaders with their own passions. While I've focused on brutality and the health risks of incarceration, Ross MacDonald has been leading the charge toward understanding the links between housing, addiction, and incarceration, and Elizabeth Ford is working to understand the mental health profile of our patients in a much more sophisticated manner than I ever could. The chief of our nursing service, Nancy Arias, has become a national leader in adapting electronic medical records to jail settings in a way that can detect interruptions in access to care, as well as probing the quality of care.

In preparing this book, I've relied on the stories of people who have been harmed in the NYC jail system, as well as data that we and others have published. In using information that is public, I hope to focus on the legitimacy of this argument rather than the personal experiences that I've had in various positions. I certainly have encountered ample frustrations and battles in correctional health services, and I've been on the losing side of plenty of fights. But I'm mindful of this quote from Eleanor Roosevelt: "Great minds discuss ideas; average minds discuss events; small minds discuss people." In this spirit, I will include a few anecdotes in this book that reflect some realities in the jail system, but not as means to settle scores or insult anyone.

Documenting the health risks of incarceration will not fix these problems. But in taking honest stock of these risks and how they reflect the functioning of the jail systems, not the failings of a few individuals, we can hopefully end some of our shared delusions about mass incarceration. There are currently about 3,000 jails and 2,000 prisons in the United States. Jails hold people awaiting trial (mostly there because they cannot afford bail) and those serving short sentences, usually of a year or less. Prisons hold people whose cases are completed and who are serving sentences of more than a year. But among the approximately 12 million incarcerations that occur each year in the United States, over 90 percent occur in jails. Because jails are chaotic and concealed from outside view, we only become aware of them when very bad outcomes occur, such as deaths. As a result, our periodic glimpses into this area miss the systemic failings of the systems we've designed, and we make the repeated error of blaming individuals for outcomes that we've essentially predetermined. Some of the stories in this book involve horrible, even criminal acts by jail staff, and their punishment is certainly warranted. But for most patients who pass through jail, the health consequences of their incarceration go well beyond the actions of one or even several staff. Correctional officers suffer some of the worst consequences of our jail system. They're often thrown into dehumanizing dynamics with inmates and either disbelieved or not listened to when they relate the grim realities of what they face. Virtually every press release in the wake of these tragedies is the same, stating that the sheriff or commissioner has zero tolerance for any misconduct and that the actions of a few do not reflect the rest of the staff. Almost never do we read that the outcome reflects the design of the jail system or the pipeline that leads people to be incarcerated.

One of the universal features of the jail setting is tribalism. The correctional officers look out for each other, as do the inmates and the health staff. These groups cooperate and coexist in many ways, but at times of conflict or friction, their allegiance is often to each other rather than a greater good. The fault lines between these groups reflect more than different philosophies; they're a result of the design of the jail system, which pits one group's interests against those of another. The more I work in the jails, the more I see the daily frustrations that everyone inside contends with and how weak leadership can allow these natural responses to real threats to produce animosity toward another group. Political leaders will often urge the various groups to get along or at least refrain from public conflict, which usually results in the weakest of the groups (the inmates and health staff) being told to keep quiet about their problems. But this doesn't mean that the concerns of security staff are addressed either. When the approach to governance is to avoid bad news, poorly designed systems like jails are bound to produce bad outcomes. Some of these problems are much worse at Rikers than at other jails I'm familiar with in the United States, especially the violence and sexual assault. But I have been to quite a few "model" facilities where there's little violence and the health and security staff are in lockstep, but where seriously mentally ill patients are kept quiet, are locked in cells, and receive perpetual involuntary medication, with little external oversight.

The resistance to transparency in jails isn't just a product of the paramilitary nature of the setting. It's also tied into the role of litigation in improving jail conditions. For better or worse, most improvements in health care for the incarcerated have come as a result of litigation, starting with the case that established a right to health care for the incarcerated, *Estelle v. Gamble*, in 1976. From that case until today our nation has relied on lawyers and judges to promote better care (and less harm) for the incarcerated. This approach has many flaws and attributes, but it's important to grasp when considering the resistance to transparency among wardens, sheriffs, and other officials. Then add in the almost-universal design of having all health care locally funded, designed, and overseen by security staff, and the health risks of incarceration become more predictable. Unfortunately, the cycle of neglect and abuse in jails followed by investigation, outrage, and court involvement is fairly routine. Almost all the large jails in the United States have been subject to multiple investigations and court settlements with the DOJ or class action plaintiffs, and the only surprise is whether the topic is poor health care, brutality, or other conditions of confinement. Overall, this can seem like a pretty bleak set of problems to try to improve.

I OFTEN COMPARE THIS LANDSCAPE to what my father encountered as a pediatrician in the late 1960s. He and a group of other pediatricians, social workers, and law enforcement professionals became deeply disturbed in caring for children who had been repeatedly abused by family members. At the time, pets had more legal protections than children, so he and a group of other pediatricians and lawyers met in Colorado in 1970 and devised a strategy to use their partnerships to criminalize physical abuse of children.[9] Shortly thereafter, a 6-month-old boy was brought to my father's hospital with multiple injuries to his head and torso. The boy's father reported that he had fallen about two feet from his crib to the floor, but my father noted fractures to his skull and ribs, and a lumbar puncture revealed blood in the cerebrospinal fluid, indicating brain hemorrhage. These injuries were completely inconsistent with the account given by the father, who did note that he had been frustrated with the infant's crying. Tragically, the boy died the next morning. My father documented his findings and worked with local police and prosecutors to testify concerning the intentional nature of this boy's injuries. This case became the first in Minnesota to establish "battered child syndrome," which set a path for other states to follow suit.[10] While the problem of child abuse is ongoing, and the efforts to address it predated the efforts of my father and his colleagues, I'm nonetheless struck that there was a real change in the consciousness of the country. In the mid-1960s, child abuse was an unspoken shame. By the 1980s, it was accepted as a felony, and the disciplines of medicine, social work, education, and law enforcement were essentially in agreement on the importance of the issue, with public support. When I compare my dad's mission to mine, I think that our patients in jail are viewed less sympathetically than young children, and the abuser of our patients is a network of governmental institutions, not individual family members. Nonetheless, the role of health professionals in calling out the harms to patients always requires partnerships outside our discipline to have an impact. Also, taking up the cause of protecting our patients is a very rewarding career despite all the frustrations that come with it.

Decreasing the health risks of incarceration requires addressing problems behind bars, but it also requires less incarceration. This is an area where NYC is far ahead of most large cities. In the past 20 years, the number of people held in the NYC jail system has been cut by more than half, from a daily population of over 21,000 under Mayor Rudolph Giuliani to about 9,000 in 2018. During a roughly equivalent period, the Los Angeles County jail census fell by about 30 percent, whereas the Chicago, Houston, and Philadelphia jail populations stayed essentially the same or increased.[11] During this time, hundreds of new jails were built in the United States, and the overall rate of incarceration more than doubled. The success of NYC should represent a standard for the rest of the nation to follow, but it also underscores the point of this book. Even as NYC has come up with innovative alternatives to incarceration, the health risks of being in the jails have continued and, in many cases, worsened. The amount of money spent on the jails, the number of correctional officers, the health staff and budget—all of these have increased over the past 20 years, despite a falling daily population. So even if the rest of the nation follows the example of NYC in correcting mass incarceration, there is a risk that they will also replicate our failings in how the incarcerated are treated.

Even with massive diversion of people away from jails, we will still have millions of Americans passing through these settings every year. So against the wishes of many, we need to both reduce the rates of incarceration and invest in more humane and effective practices inside jails. We have charged jails with a job they simply cannot do. Sheriffs are not health administrators, correction officers are not social workers, and jail cells are not hospital rooms. And even when the appropriate resources are present in a jail to provide medical care, the staff are influenced by the security services in ways that harm patients. This book documents the ways in which these poorly designed systems confer new health risks on the incarcerated, as well as opportunities for reducing those risks. We should expect that people in jail will receive their medications or have access to health services. We should also expect that rape and violence are not accepted features of going to jail. But to get to that point will require not only significant financial investment in jails but also a commitment to redesign and transparency. In NYC, this will also require closing Rikers Island and likely opening another jail in the community. The NYC jail system consists of a complex of nine jails on Rikers Island, as well as three jails in the boroughs of Manhattan, the Bronx, and Brooklyn. The pitfalls of operating an inaccessible island colony of jails goes well beyond abuse and neglect, as the jails on Rikers are falling apart and visiting detainees is a thoroughly humiliating and enraging experience for families and friends. These reforms will be resisted by many, including jailers, politicians, and advocates, all for different reasons. Still, our obligation is to develop a smarter and more just approach to incarceration, and one of the first steps must be revealing just how these settings cause harm to detainees. Without an honest sense of how jail creates health risks, we will continue to undervalue alternatives to incarceration and resist prison reforms.

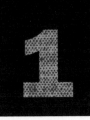

Dying in Jail

Carlos Mercado and Angel Ramirez

CARLOS MERCADO DIED A DEATH of pure neglect. He was a 45-year-old with diabetes, and when he told officers in the jail intake that he was sick and needed insulin, they told him he was withdrawing from drugs and gave him a garbage bag to vomit into. Many months after his death, surveillance video surfaced of Mr. Mercado's final hours in the jail. In this video, Mr. Mercado is seen falling down, clutching a garbage bag full of his own vomit, and laying on the jail floor. Security staff went about their work, literally stepping over him as he lay dying. All these events took place a short distance from the insulin he needed.

The most serious health risk of incarceration is death. Like Mr. Mercado, hundreds more men and women die every year as a result of something that happens to them in jail or prison. The cause is usually portrayed as individual negligence of health or security staff, but in truth, these examples reveal a constant risk of incarceration, a feature of the system we have designed and grown accustomed to.

Carlos Mercado was arrested in Brooklyn on a drug charge and brought to the biggest and most chaotic of the jails on Rikers Island, the Anna M. Kross Center (AMKC). When Mr. Mercado stepped off the bus, he would have come into a part of the jail called intake, where detainees are shuttled through a series of chaotic pens that can hold 20 to 40 people standing, sitting, or lying down. As correction officers search newly arrived detainees, make their jail identification tags, and complete other tasks, people move from pen to pen, until they are done with their security intake and can cross the hall for their medical intake. The intake areas are known to be violent, chaotic, and difficult to manage since large numbers of people are crammed into small pens. In addition to the general stress of ending up in jail, some people are going into withdrawal from drugs and alcohol, while others are actively getting high from drugs they have on them or get in the pens. In this particular jail, AMKC, many people were in the midst of opiate withdrawal, or "dope sick," during intake, which would color officers' response to Mr. Mercado's medical emergency.

We know quite a bit about Mr. Mercado's final hours through official reports, as well as considerable press coverage.[1] The official report into his death, although redacted, includes considerable information about what other inmates saw, as well as the review of video and interviews with security staff. The report notes that video shows Mr. Mercado arriving in the AMKC intake at about 7:00 p.m., walking on his own from the first to third pen. About two hours later, the other inmates in the third pen come out to be counted, but not Mr. Mercado. After another two hours, an officer opens the pen door, and Mr. Mercado is seen on video falling out of the doorway onto the jail floor, rolling back and forth. At this time Mr. Mercado appears unable to get up and places a shirt under his head, while more than one officer steps over him as they pass. Several minutes later, correction officers assist Mr. Mercado, who appears unsteady, back into the pen. About 30 minutes later, the other people in the third pen come out to eat, but not Mr. Mercado. Shortly afterward, at about 12:30 a.m., Mr. Mercado exits the pen holding a bag full of liquid, his own vomit. By 2:00 a.m., Mr. Mercado's movements on video show him stumbling, breathing heavily, and stooped over. By this time, Mr. Mercado has progressed through the various intake pens and is near the last pen before being taken to medical. By 4:45 a.m., correctional staff are seen bringing a mop and bucket to Mr. Mercado's pen, though he is still inside. At about 6:30 a.m., Mr. Mercado exits the pen with the bag full of vomit, leans against the wall, and crosses the hallway to medical for his intake examination.

The actual cause of Mr. Mercado's death was a condition called diabetic ketoacidosis. This emergency occurs when patients lack insulin in their blood supply, which is required to push sugar into the cells of their organs and tissues. As cells become energy starved, the body cannibalizes its fat stores, also producing waste products known as ketoacids. If enough ketoacids build up, patients can die. Patients with diabetes, especially those who take insulin, are pretty knowledgeable about needing to keep their blood sugar in balance, but diabetic ketoacidosis is such an emergency that fast access to emergency care is critical. One patient reported the following about diabetic ketoacidosis: "You are hot. You are freezing. You are confused. You are blacked out but coherent. You go to talk but words fail you. Time flies and goes in slow motion simultaneously. You will likely smell and look like death."[2] This same patient made her way to the hospital with her husband and reported, "Thankfully, I vomited shortly after entering, which prompted the care team to triage me in advance of the full waiting room. . . . I remember the doctor saying, had we waited 30 minutes more, I would be in a coma. I remember waking up in the ICU [Intensive Care Unit] with a doctor telling me I was lucky to be alive."

This report came from a patient in the community who had access to hospital care with medically trained staff and a spouse at her side to advocate for her. Mr. Mercado's experience while suffering the exact same medical emergency was quite different. Interviews with the other men who were around Mr. Mercado during his time at AMKC reveal that he was asking for help and feeling sick throughout his journey from pen to pen. Several stated that he was given a garbage bag to vomit into, that he told multiple officers that he was diabetic and needed medical attention, and that he was told "no, you're just withdrawing." One witness reported that he thought Mr. Mercado vomited 10–20 times, while another reported that a correctional officer said, "Well if he don't get up when I call him, he ain't gonna get his methadone." Mr. Mercado was then "walked" across the hallway to yet another pen to wait for his health intake. There, he was briefly seen by one health staff member while awaiting his medical intake encounter, but he died shortly thereafter. This delay in his medical assessment was another critical error and was identified in both the oversight report and another press report.[3]

ALMOST EVERY DEATH like Mr. Mercado's is immediately labeled a tragedy or failure of a small number of individuals. Certainly there were glaring problems with how specific individuals acted in Mr. Mercado's case. Any person in jail or prison should be able to report needing medical care and receive it for emergencies. And having difficulty standing and vomiting are certainly serious-enough problems that every jail and prison should expect staff to immediately call medical staff or report it as a medical emergency. All of these requirements are detailed in the job requirements for correctional officers and the various laws that govern local jails and prisons. Shortly before Mr. Mercado's death, we had published a review of a decade of jail deaths in New York City, which showed a dramatic fall in the death rate over that time period, largely driven by the introduction of effective treatments for HIV.[4] This was the period during which our health service developed a dedicated HIV program, which included a team of HIV treatment adherence counselors and a set of policies and procedures to connect patients with their medications as soon as they entered jail. But despite doing a better job with HIV and medical care overall during this time, our numbers revealed another important statistic: the share of all deaths that were unnatural (homicide, suicide, or accident) remained essentially unchanged, at 23.5 percent. This group represents the core of the health risks of jail. Suicide, homicide, and accidental death all seem quite different, but they share a strong linkage to failures inside the jail system. The inability to identify people with risks for suicide is a failure of the correctional health and security services. So is the inability to safeguard incarcerated people from being beaten to death by other inmates or correction officers or dying from lack of insulin.

That reduction in overall death in the jails obscured an important subset of deaths like Mr. Mercado's: those caused by actions taken inside the walls of the facility. Around the time Mr. Mercado died, I started tracking this subset of deaths with my staff, and we termed them "jail-attributable" deaths. Jail-attributable deaths included suicides, homicides, and many of the early-admission deaths like Mr. Mercado's where systemic or individual errors made a substantial contribution to the patient's death. In the years between when we started this tracking and my departure, jail-attributable deaths usually represented 10 to 20 percent of all deaths in a given year, with medical deaths from preexisting or acute conditions being the most common reason for death. There were a few years where the share of jail-attributable deaths rose to half or more, and many of the cases that drove those spikes are included in this book. The label of "jail-attributable death" is one we created to explain our own data, but it is not used by other correctional health systems or by the US Department of Justice in tracking deaths in custody. It should be. We need a way to look past the raw number of deaths in jails to make an apples-to-apples comparison of how often jails are contributing to the death of people in their custody. Mr. Mercado's death could be chalked up to the neglect of a few staff members, but his was only one of several jail-attributable deaths in this same AMKC hallway over a four-year period.

Two years before Carlos Mercado would suffer and die in the intake pens of AMKC, Angel Ramirez came into the same jail intake after being arrested for drug possession. During his medical intake, Mr. Ramirez was found to be in the midst of alcohol withdrawal and directed by health staff into a dorm for patients being treated for alcohol and/or opiate withdrawal. We called this housing area the "double detox dorm," and it was a critical spot for the health service because we could bring nurses twice daily to check each patient for symptoms of withdrawal, give out medications to prevent worsening withdrawal, and decide who needed hospital transfer. Two days later, Mr. Ramirez's condition worsened, but we didn't know, because when nurses came to the unit to check everyone, he wasn't there.

Many people entering jail or prison are dealing with some sort of substance withdrawal, and alcohol withdrawal is the one most commonly fatal. Heavy drinkers will often feel sick when they stop cold turkey, with moderate withdrawal involving the "shakes." The expression "the DTs" (delirium tremens) refers to the bizarre set of hallucinations and behaviors that sometimes accompany more serious alcohol withdrawal. References to seeing pink elephants and giant snakes and spiders are right on target, and these hallucinations can be accompanied by wild fluctuations in blood pressure and heart rate, seizures, and death. The treatment for acute withdrawal is hospitalization with very close monitoring of vital signs and treatment with drugs called benzodiazepines (like Ativan or Librium) to reduce these symptoms. In reviewing patient accounts of DTs, I came across this post from a patient to a health blog: "After two days I was mentally out of it with an increasing heart rate. By day three I was hallucinating, had head butted a doctor, had kicked my wife, and was lashed to my bed. The doctor told my wife that both pancreatitis and the DTs could kill me, so prepare for the worst."[5]

The dorm Mr. Ramirez was transferred to was designed to treat mild alcohol and opiate withdrawal and detect more serious cases that required immediate transfer to the hospital. According to accounts of Mr. Ramirez's death, he was in line in his dorm awaiting his medicine when he started acting strangely and was pulled out of line and placed in a small area outside his housing area, out of sight of the nursing staff. While in this area, he reported to guards that "he was seeing people throwing knives at him and trains going around his bed." Having missed his evaluation and medicine, he was returned to his bed in the dorm, but he continued to act more bizarrely overnight, digging through a trash can looking for his "meth." At some point, a correction officer approached him, and he swung at the officer, resulting in a single, quick body blow from the officer, knocking down Mr. Ramirez and ending the situation. The day of his death, I would be told by senior correctional officials that this was the only physical force applied to Mr. Ramirez and that his death appeared to be a tragic but unavoidable turn of events.

At the point of this altercation with Mr. Ramirez (commonly called a use of force), all policies and procedures directed that he be taken to the jail intake to make sure he didn't have any weapons and then be promptly taken to the medical clinic for an injury evaluation. Every use of force, no matter how it started or ended, must result in the patient being taken ("produced") to the medical clinic for this encounter, a standard part of correctional policy across American jails. This process is essential not only to find and treat injuries but also to protect correctional officers by objectively documenting the lack of injuries in the immediate aftermath. But instead, Mr. Ramirez was apparently taken back to the very same AMKC intake hallway where Carlos Mercado would languish, and he was placed in a pen out of camera range and beaten by several correction officers. One witness heard Mr. Ramirez say "No mas" during this beating, while another saw a handcuffed Ramirez being struck by correction officers "with nightsticks coming down hard." That witness wrote, "This was not just a homicide. It was a cold, heartless, corrupt murder."[6] Somehow in this process, correction officers put Mr. Ramirez into a fresh jumpsuit and dragged him to the medical clinic, where he was dropped off without mention of his injuries, let alone how they were sustained. After medical evaluation, he was transferred to the hospital, but he died shortly thereafter. The autopsy the next day revealed a large amount of blood in Mr. Ramirez's abdomen, multiple rib fractures, and a lacerated spleen, all evidence of a fatal beating. Nobody was ever charged with a crime in Mr. Ramirez's case, and many of the facts of this horrible beating only became known to us in the health service after Jake Pearson of the Associated Press reported them. In both Mr. Mercado's and Mr. Ramirez's cases, a medical problem was misinterpreted by security staff, leading to abuse for one, neglect for the other, but ultimately death for both men. There is no doubt that individual staff members bear responsibility for these and similar deaths by denying an obviously ill patient medical care. However, it is the failure of systems that makes space for these mistakes and abuses.

Mr. Mercado and Mr. Ramirez are far from the only people who died as a result of being in jail during my time at Rikers. In fact, they are not even the only ones who died preventable deaths in the AMKC hallway. But understanding their deaths helps to establish that going to jail can mean dying, through no fault of the incarcerated. In epidemiology, we have decades of understanding that bad outcomes like diseases or death often result from the interaction of environmental and personal risk factors. This concept has made its way into public understanding of diseases like breast cancer, autism, and heart disease but remains absent from discussions of correctional health. In the United States, because of the hidden and paramilitary nature of health care in jails and prisons and the lack of any universal standards to monitor care, we end up having the same sad discussion around every tragedy. When someone dies in jail or prison, the security service will either do its best to link the death to a personal failing by the deceased patient or chalk it up to a few bad apples when staff abuse or neglect is clearly implicated. But we have more than enough information to tease out how these settings contribute to death, and do so unevenly. As we will see with the subsequent stories, the health risks of jail are more often visited on people with behavioral health problems, people of color, women, and those who identify as LGBT. In addition, many health risks of jail like solitary confinement and injuries during use of force are tightly linked to the problem of dual loyalty, the erosion of the health service's mission to care for patients as a result of the security setting.

The easiest way to reduce the health risks of jail is to reduce incarceration. The rate of death for people in jail is higher than for people not in jail, as is the rate for those formerly incarcerated when compared to those never incarcerated. The migration of poor and minority Americans into jails and prisons, often as a result of behavioral health concerns, has pushed our nation into a downward spiral. As we have built more jails, we have mandated that the paramilitary organizations that run these settings adequately screen for and treat health problems. And despite knowing that these are places where abuse and neglect are inherent to the institutional structure, we have done little to monitor for these problems and have placed almost every correctional health service under the thumb of the security service. Because security officials oversee jail health care, the scope of care remains narrow, and the transparency and quality of care remain far below what we accept in community settings; in addition, this model, for the most part, involves for-profit staffing companies. The result is that despite a fairly common and predictable set of systems, issues relating to preventable death and injury remain.

One area of incarceration-related death that is completely hidden from national reporting is overdose after release from jail or prison. Substance use disorder is the most common diagnosis in correctional health, yet virtually no treatment is provided to these patients, and our own data in NYC have revealed that their risk of death in the first weeks after release is eight times higher than that of the rest of the population.[7] Virtually every county in the United States has put together a task force of law enforcement and health officials to try to stem the tide of opiate overdose deaths. These task forces work to balance several priorities, including decreasing local supply of illegal drugs, changing prescribing practices of health providers, and assembling harm reduction and treatment options. Many of these activities are funded in part or entirely via forfeitures of cash and assets relating to drug arrests, so this national response to our addiction problems is partly wedded to doing more of what has failed—criminalization. Many cities and counties have struck a balance by creating drug courts that can steer people toward treatment instead of incarceration. But like sheriffs and commissioners of correction, many judges and prosecutors insist on ineffective abstinence-only 28-day treatment programs because they don't approve of the most evidence-based treatments, methadone and buprenorphine.[8] Methadone and buprenorphine are medicines that people take every day, yet they don't cure them of their addiction. In fact, quick fixes for addiction are extremely rare, and when people are cycled in and out of quick abstinence-only programs, the result is many people facing the same risk of fatal overdose just after they finish their program, as well as, of course, the continuation of "need" and funding for these programs. Furthermore, as people are steered into ineffective treatments as part of their drug court agreements, every "failure" is a new opportunity for incarceration. The unfortunate reality is that addiction, especially to heroin, is a lifelong struggle for many and that the path to recovery is long and often includes relapse. The goals, however, are to keep people alive, help them get and keep a job, offer housing support, and help them maintain their family and social networks. These are the elements that can support a long-term life without drugs, but changing a person's social context is a decades-long journey, and certainly not achievable in 28 days. The knowledge that rates of overdose death spike just after release from jail and prison should push us to jail fewer people for drug-related offenses and also to adopt evidence-based treatments inside jail, but the connection between incarceration and these deaths seems to have eluded much of the nations' opiate overdose discussion.

Not only does forcing people into withdrawal from opiates cause unnecessary pain and suffering; it also drives preventable deaths. At Rikers, patients can receive methadone and buprenorphine, but unfortunately it's one of the only US jails where that is the case. For Mr. Mercado, the delay in being seen by health staff meant that his medical emergency was treated as simply being "dope sick." Methadone and buprenorphine are thought of as effective agents to reduce overdose death but are also associated with lower all-cause mortality for the incarcerated. In Australia, a 22-year study of methadone usage among persons with criminal justice involvement found that there was a 94 percent reduction in risk of death from any cause in the first four weeks of prison, which is very relevant to discussion of jail deaths.[9] Also, I think we need to reassess the idea that opiate withdrawal is not fatal, especially in jail. We have a high percentage of patients in jail who have both chronic opiate use and also liver cirrhosis from hepatitis C or alcohol use. These people are at high risk for catastrophic bleeding in the blood vessels of the GI tract, and I have seen numerous cases of forced opiate withdrawal causing the predictable signs of vomiting and retching, followed by a new and fatal bleeding in the blood vessels of the upper GI tract.

But even if we do achieve some dismantling of mass incarceration, there will be millions of incarcerations each year in the United States. We still have 9,000 New Yorkers locked up on any given day, representing about 50,000 incarcerations a year. In the United States, incarcerations—a total of about 11 million and 1 million each year in jail and prison, respectively—can be dramatically reduced, but they will never be eliminated. Hence, we need to commit to reducing the risk of death behind bars. This book explores the evidence to find ways in which we can identify and reduce the health risks of jail, but we need to start by acknowledging that incarceration brings a risk of death, as it did for Mr. Mercado and Mr. Ramirez. Once we agree on this simple point, we should then compel every jail and prison to track and report their death data, including jail-attributable deaths, alongside other, more common health outcomes such as injuries, overdose, and medication interruptions (table A.2). Fortunately, the passage of recent legislation has forced jails and prisons to start reporting on one health risk, sexual assault. If we don't start with an acknowledgment that incarceration carries a risk of death, then we fail the patients who die in these settings, but we also miss out on a compelling reason to reduce incarceration.

EVEN AFTER SOMEONE DIES while incarcerated, the prison system continues to color medical assessment by influencing how medical examiners characterize deaths. In some cases, local sheriffs have intimidated or threatened medical examiners just for doing their job. One recent report involved a sheriff calling a medical examiner with a threat to get the physician's license revoked for investigating two deaths in the Milwaukee County Jail. One death involved a patient who died of a seizure, and correctional officers are alleged to have picked him up and dropped him on his head because they thought he was faking his seizure. The other death involved a patient with behavioral health problems who reportedly died of dehydration after being locked in his cell and having the water shut off.[10]

The methods used to exonerate security services from death may rely on pseudoscience as much as overt threats. One example is the nonspecific term "excited delirium." The essence of excited delirium is that someone with acute drug intoxication or other unclear agitation acts wildly, physically struggles (with law enforcement), and dies. This is not a recognized diagnosis or cause of death, but it has taken root in classifying jail and other law enforcement deaths. The origins of excited delirium can be traced back to Bell's mania in 1849, but the modern description includes "acute behavioral disinhibition manifested in a cluster of behaviors that may include bizarreness, aggressiveness, agitation, ranting, hyperactivity, paranoia, panic, violence, public disturbance, surprising physical strength, profuse sweating due to hyperthermia, respiratory arrest, and death." The most consistent feature of excited delirium deaths seems to be contact with law enforcement, not any specific and consistent pathological cause of death such as cardiac arrhythmia, asphyxia, or seizure.[11] Medical examiners sometimes use the label of excited delirium, but it is not accepted by most physicians' organizations, and it is not in the *ICD-10*, the official list of medical diagnoses we rely on in medicine. Aside from this term being used almost exclusively to describe law enforcement–related deaths, another telltale sign of the lack of precision behind "excited delirium" is the shifting set of physiologic causes attributed to it over time. This collection of symptoms was initially attributed to acute cocaine intoxication in the 1980s, but then it morphed into a description of symptoms during deaths involving Tasers in the 2000s.[12] Although there has been one book written on this topic, much more research is needed, including the prospect for racial disparity in its use. Later, in discussion of racial disparities, I will describe another racially targeted diagnosis, drapetomania.[13] Drapetomania was a mental health diagnosis created in the 1800s to describe slaves running away from their plantation or owner. Like excited delirium, drapetomania was useful in ascribing a pathology to the person harmed instead of the group inflicting the harm.

Establishing transparency about death in jail is a critical first step to reducing this and other health risks. Mr. Mercado's and Mr. Ramirez's deaths were preventable, and although there is some overall reporting of deaths in jails and prisons to the DOJ, there is no scrutiny of preventable deaths. The subset of deaths that we tracked as "jail-attributable" stem more from the jail setting than from the patients, including deaths from withdrawal, trauma, suicide, and diabetic ketoacidosis. Overall, these types of deaths appear to represent about one-fourth to one-third of jail deaths, and the DOJ or the Centers for Disease Control and Prevention should facilitate mandatory reporting of rates of these types of deaths across all jail settings. Looking at the rate of all death and then preventable death by facility would allow for fair comparisons of this outcome in jails across size, location, and demographic profile. It would also allow for analysis of deaths based on type of health service, including those that are independent, those that are controlled by the security service, and those that use for-profit staffing companies. When I looked at a decade of deaths in immigration detention facilities, I paid special attention to the rate of suicide in a subset of for-profit detention centers.[14] This type of analysis should be public and automatic for our nation's jails.

A second avenue to reduce the risk of death in jail is to initiate earlier contact between health staff and our patients. In the case of Mr. Mercado, he languished for hours in the jail intake, with his requests for medicine being ignored. Since his death, we have worked with the Department of Correction to bring health staff into the intake corridor so we can initiate our intake encounter earlier, but the long-standing practice of keeping injured patients in the jail intakes for several hours without notifying health staff continues. In my final weeks at Rikers we continued to find patients who were forgotten about in these intake pens, and the problem is so pervasive that most jails actually have a pen known to all as the "forget about me" or "why me" pen.

Another way to mitigate the health risks in jail is to see the patients before they arrive in jail. Recently, we have moved our initial contact with patients out into the central booking of Manhattan, before the bail decision has been made. Anyone arrested in NYC is taken to a central booking station at one of four courthouses, where they receive a brief health screen by an emergency medical technician working for the NYC Fire Department several hours before they see a judge and bail is decided. This screen occurs on paper and doesn't link to any actions in the jail regarding triage of the intake encounter. We had long aspired to replace this quick screen that occurs on paper with a health screen done by our staff in correctional health, and after years of efforts with the NYC Police Department, we finally succeeded in getting support to take over this function in Manhattan. We developed a web-based application that converts key variables from the nursing screening done by our nursing staff into red flags that can trigger expedited intake.[15] I left correctional health before this pre-arraignment screening could be scaled up, but aside from allowing earlier health contact for jail-bound persons, it provides a second critical promise, to identify persons who can be diverted away from jail toward health and housing services before the bail decision is made.

The third critical requirement to reduce preventable death in jail is the development of a legitimate information management system. This wonky-sounding issue comes down to knowing where every patient/inmate is at any time and how long they have been there. For Mr. Mercado, sitting in the intake pens for hours was a fatal error. In the case of Mr. Ramirez, the officers who beat him to death in the jail intake relied on their ability to move him into that pen and keep him there as long as they wanted. If the jails had an information management system akin to emergency departments, all patients in the intake area would have their time in the area displayed on a dashboard, along with their reason for being there, their next step, and any critical information like suicide watch, hospital return, and so on. This lack of transparency creates a lack of accountability that can be seen in injuries, sexual abuse, and many of the health risks of jail.

Carlos Mercado and Angel Ramirez both died soon after arriving on Rikers Island, and they died *because* they were in jail. Mr. Mercado pleaded for medical attention but only got a garbage bag to vomit in while he slipped into a fatal complication of his diabetes. Mr. Ramirez was identified as experiencing potentially fatal alcohol withdrawal by health staff when he arrived at the same jail. He was placed in a special unit for people being treated for this exact condition, which often includes wild and bizarre behavior. When he acted up, he was restrained by security staff and taken back to the jail intake, where he was beaten to death.

Not all people who die while in jail or prison died because they were incarcerated, but many do. In these cases, a preventable death is often blamed on a health problem of the patient or, at most, the errors of a few individuals. The cases of Carols Mercado and Angel Ramirez reveal how preventable death is a systemic risk of incarceration. Data from our own work, as well as from other jails and prisons, show that a significant percentage of deaths behind bars are preventable, and therefore we should treat incarceration as a risk factor for death, just like smoking or obesity. Until death and other health risks are properly ascribed to incarceration, we perpetuate the myth that bad outcomes in these settings are the fault of the incarcerated or a few bad apples among staff.

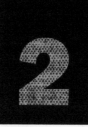

Injury and Violence

I N THE MOST VIOLENT and notorious of the 12 New York City jails, Robert Hinton was hog-tied by correctional officers, taken into a cell, and beaten until the bones in his face and neck were broken. Just before this beating, as Mr. Hinton was being led to his cell, he feared that a beating was coming once he was out of camera range. So he did maybe the most natural thing one could imagine: he sat down. Several minutes later, after a mysterious failure of the unit's cameras, Mr. Hinton was inside his cell, grievously injured. Mr. Hinton's story reveals how the risk for injury and violence in jail can flow from the jail itself, not just the people held there. As a 26-year-old inmate, Robert Hinton was considered a security threat in the jails because of a purported affiliation with the Bloods gang and his criminal record, including attempted murder. For interactions with Mr. Hinton, higher levels of security were used, including extra officers to assist with movement and enhanced restraints such as leg irons and waist chains. These measures, designed to reduce the potential for Mr. Hinton to harm others, made it relatively easy for a group of six officers to take him into a cell and beat him. Although I was shocked by the extent of Mr. Hinton's injuries, they fit a pattern that I had seen in 2012 and 2013, in which serious injuries occurred during interactions with correctional officers. As a result, I worked with our doctors, nurses, and information technology team to dig into this problem, including sophisticated data analyses and more thorough assessments of individual patients who had poorly explained injuries. The result would be several new sources of data on brutality in the NYC jails, including a report on the epidemiology of the use of force by Department of Correction officers, which identified common types and victims of violent abuse, supporting the nascent efforts of the US Department of Justice on this very issue.

On the day in question, Mr. Hinton was being escorted into the Mental Health Assessment Unit for Infracted Inmates (MHAUII) when he and another officer apparently recognized each other from prior altercations and exchanged words. Quickly, the number of officers surrounding Mr. Hinton grew from two to five. As he was being led down the cellblock toward his cell, Mr. Hinton sat down and refused to advance. The walkway portion of the cellblock is on camera, while the area inside the cells is off camera. This limitation is used by staff and patients alike to strike at, spit on, or otherwise abuse someone off camera while maintaining appropriate behavior on camera. I have cared for patients who reported not only refusing to go into their cells, for fear of being beaten, but also actually trying to run or crawl out of their cells to get on camera while being beaten, only to be pulled back into the cell. Inmates looking to assault officers could turn the tables, going into their cells willingly and then striking officers when off camera. In the case of Mr. Hinton, the 30 seconds of video just after he stopped walking disappeared. If you find that suspicious, you are not alone, but this is not the last story of this book that will involve a disappearance of video that could implicate correctional officers. As he sat, officers hog-tied Mr. Hinton, and then they carried him to his cell and reportedly beat him for approximately 10 minutes. The officers wore leather gloves to protect their hands, though gloves are banned. The account of the officers was that after being hog-tied and carried passively into his cell, Mr. Hinton then sprang up when uncuffed and put one of them in a chokehold and attacked the other four officers. From this melee, Mr. Hinton and the officers emerged with very different sets of injuries. Mr. Hinton sustained multiple lacerations and contusions to his face and head and broken bones in his nose and neck. The officers sustained some muscle strain, with one of them requiring Tylenol but nothing more.

While the beating in his cell is the dramatic aspect of this case, there are other important aspects of Mr. Hinton's story. After he was hog-tied by the officers, he was picked up by the arms and legs and basically dragged across the floor and down the stairs to his cell. Aside from injuries due to the trauma this involves, there's a small but important group of deaths associated with this type of restraint, sometimes termed "positional asphyxiation."[1]

The common features are restraint of the upper extremities and often pressure on the chest when officers sit or lay on top of someone. Especially for people with heart or lung disease, restraint combined with pressure on the chest can be deadly. These types of deaths have been well documented in jail and prison settings, as well as with police and during ambulance transport.[2] In 2014, members of the NYC Police Department were attempting to arrest Eric Garner on a sidewalk when he died in similar fashion. Mr. Garner was seen on video stating that he could not breathe, and the medical examiner found that physical pressure on his chest during the arrest played a significant role in his death.[3] Mr. Hinton sat down and refused to move, while Mr. Garner was standing and refusing to comply with orders to be handcuffed, but neither was posing a threat to law enforcement officers. Restraint is necessary in some cases, but in the instance of a person who simply refuses to move or comply with an order, there are many other options, not the least of which is to sit and talk for a few minutes. In my experience with similar circumstances with patients across the jails, although talking through a crisis didn't always fix the immediate problem, it almost never made things worse. One of my teachers in this respect was DOC deputy warden John Gallagher. I've responded to many cells, pens, and other far-flung sites with him, and his ability to take a calm and reassuring tone with a person who felt like they had gone past the point of no return has saved countless injuries and trauma. His skills in this area, as well as similar experiences in community police departments, served as a model for teams we would develop in multiple jails, called Crisis Intervention Teams (CITs). It would take us another two years to get the attention of city hall on this issue, but eventually we would train CITs of correctional officers and health staff who could respond to just this type of incident with the goal of de-escalation.

We know quite a bit about Mr. Hinton's injuries because they were made public during the disciplinary trial of officers involved in the beating.[4] This highlights another structural component of jail abuse: the power of correctional officers and their unions to steer almost all cases of reported physical and sexual abuse into the pathway of workplace discipline. This misdirection allows for workplace reprimand or suspension in response to acts that would land the rest of us in a criminal court. In Mr. Hinton's case, however, the judge involved in his oath trial (the official name for these disciplinary hearings) was particularly outraged at what she learned. The judgment against the officers involved in Mr. Hinton's assault came two-and-a-half years after his beating. Judge Tynia Richard recommended that the officers be fired, including one captain who had a history of many serious uses of force. By the time her decision was made, the tidal wave of press coverage and DOJ investigation had taken hold, and, almost without precedent, the officers were fired by the new DOC commissioner, Joe Ponte. As with so many before him, Robert Hinton sued NYC for the abuse he suffered and won a settlement against the city for $450,000 in September 2015. He had served a short sentence in the state prison system after being at Rikers, and then he returned home to live in Brooklyn with his mother in 2014. Shortly before he was to collect the city's settlement, he was killed, shot in the head as he visited relatives in Brownsville, Brooklyn.[5] Before his death, Robert Hinton had experienced a decade of repeated incarcerations. His time in Rikers was violent and chaotic. Many have presented Mr. Hinton's life as a symbol of the victimization that Rikers visits on the detained, while others see him as the perfect example of the dangerousness of the people who are held in jail. What's clear is that the interaction between Mr. Hinton and the jail system produced high levels of violence, which did more than break his neck and nose; it debased the officers involved and got them fired, and it cost NYC $450,000 and countless extra resources in treating his many injuries.

MR. HINTON'S INJURIES during this particular use of force occurred in 2012, a couple years into our concerted analysis of the rates of injuries among our patients. Our efforts to track injuries developed in a few stages, starting in 2010. That year, we collected and analyzed about 4,000 of the paper injury reports that are filled out by health and security staff after every injury visit. We found that most of the injuries were intentional and that the most common cause of injury (40% of them) was inmate fight, which wasn't a real shock. We were surprised, however, that the second-leading cause, "slip and fall," accounted for 27 percent of the cases.[6] Like most physicians who work in jails, I have seen many patients with injuries that weren't consistent with their account of what happened, often involving slipping and falling into a broken nose or jaw. As we shared these findings with DOC leadership, we also worked on developing more precise methods of injury surveillance. Because of the robust IT team we have, we were able to modify our electronic medical record (EMR) to capture information about injuries in a way that allowed us to report outcomes back to DOC more routinely. We devised an approach that had the doctors and physician assistants click on drop-down menus to gather specific variables relating to the injury and to the patient who was injured. For example, the provider would click through questions about whether the injury was intentional, who caused the injury, where in the jail it occurred, and whether there was a blow to the head. Already present in each patient's record were other critical variables like age and mental health diagnosis. In this way, we designed the clinical tool used by physicians and physician assistants to yield data we could aggregate on the profile of injuries, the injured, and the causes of injuries. When this system was first developed in 2011, we saw about 1,000 injury encounters per month, with an average daily census of 14,000 in jail. In the past several years, the daily jail census has fallen below 10,000, while the number of these encounters has risen to about 2,400 per month. Once this surveillance system was created, we would run reports of all these injury encounters to show DOC leadership which jails had the highest rates of injury during use of force, including those that involved blows to the head. In theory, a blow to the head should be rare during uses of force because of the extensive training and equipment that law enforcement officers utilize in these situations. However, our data revealed just the opposite. One of the overlaps between our clinical concerns and the interests of US Attorney Preet Bharara's investigation a couple of years later was the problem of blows to the head by security staff. Termed "head shots," these incidents should have been rare during interactions between highly trained security staff and adolescents, but our own data revealed that an adolescent was in fact more likely to sustain a blow to the head during a violent interaction with a correctional officer than during a fight with another inmate.[7]

In 2012, Mr. Hinton's injuries were part of a trend that my team and I had become alarmed about. We seemed to have more and more patients being hurt by correction officers, with many of these injuries occurring in solitary confinement. Patients held in solitary confinement who insulted, assaulted, or splashed officers (with urine, water, feces, or food) seemed to feature prominently among these use-of-force injuries. When my staff and I interviewed these patients, they would tell us that their basic access to phone, food, shower, recreation, and health care was routinely denied.

As their grievances went unaddressed, frustration would set in, and their efforts to get what they saw as basic rights would morph into lashing out in anger. Striking, insulting, or splashing an officer was a fairly reliable way to cause a response, albeit a violent one. I would later give a public report on splashing and show that 92 percent of these incidents occurred in solitary confinement units, making the point that these behaviors more accurately reflect the treatment of the incarcerated rather than criminality or mental illness.[8] Traditionally, jail managers held that there might be a few bad apples on both sides (inmates and correctional officers) and that the occasional serious injury was an unavoidable result of running a jail. But as our data piled up, it appeared as if two groups of patients were showing up repeatedly in these injury reports: adolescents and the mentally ill. In addition, it seemed that some jail settings, such as solitary confinement units and the search areas and intake pens of jails, were also overrepresented. Compounding our concern, we were also receiving troubling reports from line staff in the facilities that patients were sometimes pressured not to seek care or not to say what actually happened to them. Eventually, these reports began to shed light on the strange trend of "slip and fall" injuries we'd noticed.

One of our public health interns, Jasmine Graves, was delivering poetry and music programs to 16- to 18-year-olds, and she would occasionally relate very concerning accounts of our patients being assaulted by correctional officers. I would check the account of incidents she shared against what was recorded in our EMR. Often, it appeared as if the patient hadn't received timely or appropriate care, or may have given a completely different story to health staff. At the time, we were receiving similarly troubling accounts from other staff, from Legal Aid Society requests for care, and from family members contacting us about their loved ones. By the end of 2012, it seemed as if many of the serious injuries incurred during use of force were related to some sort of concern about access to care or the circumstances of the original injury. We'd met with DOC several times about these issues in 2011 and 2012, but without eliciting much interest on their part to investigate these matters.

Going into 2013, we decided to take a more structured approach toward the epidemiology of brutality. We committed to having one of the senior physicians review each serious injury during use of force to ensure that the appropriate care had been provided and information collected and relayed to investigators. Because of the concerns about retaliation against line staff who report abuse, we decided to see these patients personally, either myself or another member of our senior team, including the medical director, Ross MacDonald, his deputy, Zach Rosner, and our mental health director, Danny Selling.

Retaliation against health staff is a serious and pervasive problem in correctional settings. Health staff rely on correctional officers for their protection, and any animosity between these groups can result in a lack of protection for health staff. The most common type of retaliation is usually for officer(s) to suddenly become absent from their posts, leaving a health staffer alone with patients/inmates. When this happens in a high-security setting, with multiple officers watching from the safety of a command bubble, it's quite scary. Our staff have also experienced slashed tires, verbal threats, and even more colorful acts like threatening poems, dead flowers on their computers, and threatening phone calls to their cell phones, sometimes from inmates in the jail. I've experienced this a few times, but although it rattled me when a group of officers told me one Friday night in a solitary unit, "That ID badge won't protect you here," I was able to leave the building without needing their protection the very next day. The most fearless among us was always our deputy director of nursing, Colette Raspanti. Colette would make rounds in the worst intakes and housing areas across the 12 jails, and she routinely found patients who were injured or left in distress. For this work, she has likely experienced more retaliation than any of us, but she also carries a reputation of fearlessness and a high-enough rank that most officers know better than to try to intimidate her. Most officers also recognize that the work she does is as much in their interest as in the interest of patients, including the time she found officers who had accidentally locked themselves into a cell, with no means to call for help. But for the regular jail staff, who show up every day to the same shift with the same officers, these pressures are more corrosive. In the same jail where Mr. Hinton was assaulted, I once showed up asking about another patient's injures, and after I left the clinic, I was told that a high-ranking security officer strolled through the clinic yelling, "People have been talking too much!"

Because of these concerns, when we decided to see patients who had been seriously injured during interactions with DOC staff, it made sense for me and the other members of the senior team to do the evaluation. I probably saw three-fourths of these patients during Friday night sessions, when I could move around the jails more easily. During the week, I would monitor our EMR for new injuries and then review the clinical notes and the DOC injury reports that were scanned in for each incident. Every week I would find several instances in which a patient sustained serious injuries during an interaction with correctional officers, or reports that didn't involve officers but seemed suspicious, like a jaw fracture from falling on a toilet. Then, at about 5:00 pm on Fridays, I would take my list and go to the jails where these patients were being held. I always had my stethoscope around my neck, which Ross MacDonald correctly labeled as my talisman. In the 18 months or so that I did these Friday night encounters, I probably listened to only a few sets of lungs, but I always felt some small amount of protection from having that stethoscope every single time I stepped into the high-security housing areas and intake pens and cells where these injured people were being held. At the time, I was able to move around all the jails without DOC "escorting" me, so I could almost always get to the housing area where each patient was being held. Once there, I would announce myself as "medical" and confirm with the housing area officers that the patient was there, and then I would request that the patient be brought to a confidential room on the unit for evaluation. Sometimes officers refused or said they couldn't comply, but most of the time, with some waiting and politeness, I was able to see the patient. I would perform a brief physical examination when required and then tell the patient that I was going to make sure they received all of their follow-up care and also that I was going to report any allegations of abuse to both DOC and the Department of Investigation. This last part was critical because many of these patients were reporting assaults by DOC staff that had not yet been investigated. I would also tell them that if they experienced retaliation from DOC or any problems with their care, they should ask for me through the health staff, and either I or one of our senior team members would respond. Within a few weeks of starting these Friday night encounters, the inmates and DOC staff alike came to recognize that I was coming to these housing areas and intake pens for reasons that went beyond simple checkups. On some of the solitary units where abuse was rampant, patients would call my name from their cells, and correctional officers would stiffen and slow-walk my requests to see patients. In some instances, officers would outright refuse to produce patients for me to see, or tell me their side of how the patient came to be injured.

A small number of the patients I saw were injured minutes or hours before, and my role was a combination of initial care and getting an accurate story of how they were injured. If I received word of a bad injury during the week, I would go see the patient myself or ask one of our team members to go. From 2012 to 2015, we saw approximately 200 patients who were seriously injured during use of force, and in November 2013 we were able to finally pull together all the key variables about injury severity, cause of injury, and access to care. Despite the significant modifications we had made to our EMR, I still needed to do a daily review of other sources of information, such as the log of patients who were sent to the hospital or seen by our emergency medicine doctors, in order to capture all the relevant injuries. During this time, I was spending about an hour or two every day on this process of reviewing medical records, as well as two or three hours a week seeing these patients in person. We saw the same things over and over in these patient encounters, so we decided to put together a report that we could share with DOC and the Department of Investigation about what we were observing. Because our approach had become more standard as we progressed into 2013, we decided to include a total of 129 patients who were seen from January to November of that year. I shared this report widely with DOC leadership, as well as our own leadership. Although the findings of this report were immediately viewed as inflammatory, they were important to disseminate as basic information about how our patients were being injured and which patients were most at risk for serious injury, what we've called the epidemiology of brutality. This report revealed several damning trends regarding serious injury during use of force and would become a flash point when it made its way into a two-page feature in the *New York Times*.[9]

Although we had long suspected that some groups might be more likely to experience serious injury during use of force, the results of our analysis of the 129 patients were shocking. People with mental illness were twice as likely as others to end up seriously injured during use of force. Adolescent patients were three times more likely to end up seriously injured during use of force, and patients in solitary confinement four times more likely. Also, these 129 patients averaged 6.5 prior injury visits in jail, far in excess of the system-wide average we found in the original injury analysis. One of the most alarming aspects of this group was the types of injuries they sustained. Recalling that this is a cohort of people injured during use of force (e.g., interacting with professional law enforcement officers), the most common site of injury was to the face and head (73%). Most of the injuries were fractures (34%) and lacerations requiring sutures (43%). The most common fractures were to the nose, eye socket, and jaw. So Mr. Hinton's injures were not an aberration, but part of an epidemic of brutality in the NYC jail system.

Our analysis also revealed the systematic underreporting of injuries that was rampant in the NYC jails. There appeared to be two systemic flaws: some injuries were never reported, and others were reported as much less serious than they really were. The most basic issue we found in this work was that patients we saw often told us that they had been threatened with violence or solitary confinement if they told medical staff what had happened to them. In some cases, patients were even told that they would be beaten just for seeking care. Among the patients we saw for the use-of-force report, 56 percent of them reported that they had been threatened by DOC in attempts to get them to refuse care or give alternate reasons for their injuries. One young injured patient I saw had refused both X-rays and hospital transfer multiple times. Health staff continued to speak with him over the course of several days, and he slowly revealed to them that his injuries stemmed from a use of force and that the officers who injured him had threatened further beatings if he agreed to receive any medical care. Ultimately he agreed to go to the hospital, where he was found to have a jaw fracture. Another remarkable feature of this case was how he came to be injured. He reported to me that a team of correction officers came to do a cell extraction for the person in the cell next to him. Cell extractions occur when someone won't come out of their cell. Security staff assemble a team of officers in riot gear to open the cell door, rush in, and force the patient to the floor, where they are restrained and cuffed. According to this patient, when the extraction team assembled for his neighbor, he began to harangue and harass them, getting them so mad that they switched their focus completely and entered his cell and beat him.

While this patient ultimately received care, the practice of keeping patients away from our staff after use of force can cause serious harm and even death. Patients might have an injury after use of force and be kept in their cell, or they might be brought to the jail intake pens, where they could be "forgotten" for hours or days, or where they might be subject to more un-

documented violence. In these circumstances, medical staff were completely unaware of the injured patient. This denial of care (and repeated use
of force) would only come to light when a bad outcome led us or others to
examine the details of the patient's history. In one case, correctional officers
brought a gravely injured patient to a jail clinic with little information about
his injury. He was sent to the hospital but died of internal injuries just after
we saw him. When I sat with senior DOC leaders in the days after this tragedy, they gave assurances that this patient had a single use of force (the jail
term for incident with correctional officers) in his housing area, with only
a single blow to the abdomen being delivered after he attacked correctional
officers. I won't ever forget being at his autopsy and seeing the multiple liters
of blood that had filled his abdomen from this apparently magic single blow.
More than a year later, Jake Pearson from the Associated Press looked into
this case and found statements from witnesses in this jail's intake who saw
this patient brought into the area and beaten for an extended period of time
before he was put into a fresh jumpsuit and dropped at the clinic.

In addition to injuries going unreported (or reported as something other
than a use of force by a correction officer), there were many other cases where
the injury was more severe than initially stated by security officers. Injuries
in the NYC jail system were classified as A, B, or C, with A meaning serious
injury (fracture or sutures required), B meaning mild injuries requiring first
aid, and C meaning no injury. Misrepresenting injuries like this is strategic
because "upgrading" the assessment of severity was extremely difficult for
health staff to initiate and caused a higher level of scrutiny and reporting
for the security staff. As an example, a patient could be produced to the jail
clinic after a use-of-force incident, and the health staff would write on the
injury report that the patient needed an X-ray because of facial trauma. At
this point, the injury and use of force would be classified as a mild injury (B)
because there wasn't yet evidence of serious injury. It is entirely predictable
that new medical evidence would arise that required upgrading the injury
classification, much like the preliminary diagnosis given to patients in the
emergency room is often different from their diagnosis at discharge. The
critical difference is that hospitals are invested in finding the truth of a patient's injury or illness, but the NYC jail system, like many others, wanted
the opposite. Keeping the injury as a "B" was critical for jail managers because they were allowed to investigate these incidents themselves without

notification or involvement of outside agencies like the Department of Investigation. If the patient's X-ray showed a fracture, however, the injury was supposed to be classified as "A" or serious, which would prompt an external investigation into the use of force. But despite routinely needing to upgrade injuries, the DOC system for handling these cases was designed to frustrate and foil these efforts. This process could take days and required looking for the paper form that DOC used in the original incident in a central office in the jail. There was no way for us to simply say to someone in DOC that the patient's injury turned out to include a fracture and hence the injury should be considered serious.

The presence of these additional steps, combined with the frequent movement of patients from jail to jail and the disincentive of jail security staff to have more serious injuries attributed to their building, meant that this process was often simply never completed. Even more complex was the process to upgrade injuries when the patient had been hospitalized and returned many days or a week after the injury occurred. In many of these cases, patients' true injuries became known when they arrived in the jail infirmary with their hospital discharge papers, but the security staff in the jail where the injury report was initiated rarely responded to the infirmary staff about upgrading the injury. As a consequence, the inaccuracies in injury reporting seemed to be biased toward systematically underreporting the more serious injuries. Unfortunately, leadership in these jails placed tremendous pressure on managers to keep these numbers down and limit external inquiries.[10]

I learned firsthand what an uphill battle this upgrading process was when I found patients in 2013 whose injuries were obviously underreported. I often saw these patients on Friday evenings, and after examining them and reviewing their records in the EMR and the scanned copies of injury reports, I often sent an email to DOC leadership indicating that the injuries should be recorded as a serious injury because of some clinical aspect that hadn't been apparent originally. These emails would trigger a flood of responses saying that this wasn't an approved method for upgrading injuries, that the original paper form needed to be located, and, sometimes, that because I wasn't one of the dedicated doctors in the facility, I shouldn't be communicating this information. In more extreme cases, DOC would send investigators to meet with me and challenge my clinical skills and the adequacy of my physical examination. I will never forget sitting with our counsel Patrick Alberts while a DOC investigator with zero clinical training tried to poke holes in the adequacy of my physical examination of a patient's broken nose. Her challenging of my clinical assessment that a patient had suffered a nasal fracture was maddening and insulting, but had I been one of our hundreds of physician assistants or physicians, the message would have been clear: this isn't a path you want to go down. Using our clinical skills on behalf of our patients was accepted only within the limits of what the security service deemed acceptable. For a health provider who worked in the same jail clinic every day or night, this type of pushback wouldn't just be frustrating; it would come with the unspoken but very real implications of retaliation. While the barriers to getting an accurate assessment of injury severity may seem like a mix of bureaucratic tangle and the culture of violence at Rikers, this thicket of resistance is part of an effective strategy found in most jails and prisons, to hide the extent to which people are harmed by correctional officers. Compare this to how operating rooms are run in most hospitals. In addition to clear policies and redundant checks of virtually every step of an operation, any staff member in the operating room can call for a safety time-out, creating the need for the entire team to immediately address the issue. These safety time-outs are encouraged and reflect the true desire of hospitals to reduce bad outcomes during surgery.

Another striking feature of the 129 patients in our report was that 80 percent reported that they had been struck *after* being restrained, just like Mr. Hinton. As much as any other indicator, this is a hallmark of a system designed to escalate violence and bereft of any systems designed to de-escalate. There were plenty of excellent correction officers who could and did work to defuse tense situations with inmates, but the actual systems of the correction department were primarily designed to escalate. When patients became agitated or got into confrontations with each other or correction officers, the only resource available to officers was the probe team, a group of officers who would don riot gear and march to the scene of the disturbance in order to restore order. These teams have been highly effective at quelling riots, but most jail problems are not a riot, but a much smaller disturbance with critical opportunities for either escalation or de-escalation.

One core decision point is what happens when the inmates have been physically controlled. Law enforcement officers, whether in the community or in corrections, have a daunting mandate to maintain control of their environments, which sometimes requires using physical force. For police officers, a bad interaction can last a few minutes or even an hour, but when they feel goaded or provoked, they can return to their car or foot beat or office. For correctional officers, their entire shift is often spent in a housing area with 45 inmates, some of whom may harass them every day, for hours at a time. In such an unrelentingly stressful environment, turning to beatings and other abuse is a predictable consequence, but it's also a basic professional failure. This is true for the correction officer who abuses his or her power, but it is no less true of the system that fails to prevent or respond to the abuse. Striking someone after they've been restrained represents the ultimate breakdown of correctional professionalism and indicates an absent or incompetent jail management. In one well-reported incident, one of a group of young patients reportedly pushed an officer down a flight of stairs late one night. Relatively quickly, three of them were restrained. At that point the incident was essentially done. But one by one, all three were placed on gurneys, still cuffed, and taken to the medical clinic. Once wheeled into an exam cubicle (off camera), correction officers and a captain yelled at the medical staff to get in the back of the clinic, after which the beatings began. Each of the three was beaten in this manner while medical staff protested and hid in the back. When I arrived the next morning, the doctor who was assigned to the cubicle in question had started her shift by cleaning blood off the cabinets. This case never went forward as a criminal matter, because the staff who saw what happened were too scared to relate their stories. A couple of days later, I worked an overnight shift in this building, and in the middle of seeing patients, a captain who had been part of the incident approached me in my cubicle and said, "It sure was a good thing there were so many witnesses the other night." I didn't respond, and he pressed on, "So they could see that those inmates beat their own heads against the cabinets." Like any health bureaucrat, I didn't have anything snappy to say in the moment, but I rifled off an email to the Department of Investigation, the agency that is supposed to investigate wrongdoing by DOC staff. This incident also was reported to the DOJ and made its way into their report on the culture of brutality at Rikers. For me, one of the most jarring parts of this incident occurred the next morning. I arrived in the clinic and got the stories of several staff, some of whom made it clear they would not repeat their observations to others out of fear for their own safety. I sat with the one staffer who was pretty confident about reporting what she saw, and I called my boss immediately. Dr. Tom Farley, the commissioner of health, wanted to hear the firsthand account of jail staff right away, and one of the health workers on duty recounted the harrowing details of the beatings and the orders by DOC officers to move to the back of the clinic while they beat the already-restrained patients in the exam cubicle. Then she said something to Dr. Farley that revealed the normalization of abuse in jails: "I'm new here and I didn't know that when this happens, we're supposed to go in the back and stay out of the way." This staffer did end up experiencing retaliation for talking about what she observed. She was verbally harassed by DOC staff and started to receive calls from currently incarcerated patients to her cell phone. Despite our best efforts to create a safe work environment by transferring her to alternate facilities, she left her job shortly thereafter. It's also somewhat predictable that no criminal charges were ever brought in this matter. However, one of the captains involved in this incident was the same captain who directed the use of force against Robert Hinton, for which there were consequences.

Mr. Hinton's story and our data were part of raising the alarm to the rest of the city and nation about the deep problems in the NYC jail system. In January 2012, the DOJ opened an investigation into brutality by security staff against adolescent inmates. By August 2014, the DOJ concluded that the NYC DOC engaged in a pattern and practice of excessive use of force against adolescents, in violation of their constitutional rights. Around the same time, a class action lawsuit was filed by the Legal Aid Society regarding excessive force against adult inmates, and ultimately the US attorney joined the two legal processes into one. The final DOJ report, which was 79 pages long, included many references, anecdotes, and figures from our data sources and was incredibly comprehensive in its scope and depth. Several of the central findings mirrored what we had reported in our use-of-force report:

- correction officers resort to "headshots," or blows to an inmate's head or facial area, too frequently;
- force is used as punishment or retribution;
- force is used in response to inmates' verbal altercations with officers;

- use of force by specialized response teams within the jails is particularly brutal;
- correction officers attempt to justify use of force by yelling "Stop resisting!" even when the adolescent has been completely subdued or was never resisting in the first place;
- use of force is particularly common in areas without video surveillance cameras.

By 2014, most of NYC seemed in agreement that Rikers was a violent and deeply dysfunctional place, causing countless injuries to those who passed through. The job of fixing Rikers would initially fall to Joe Ponte, a longtime reformer of corrections in Maine and elsewhere. His path toward reform would be rocky and hampered by powerful people with divergent interests, including the extremely powerful Correctional Officers' Benevolent Association (COBA), led by Norman Seabrook. In my years at Rikers, it often seemed as if Norman Seabrook and COBA were more powerful than the commissioner of corrections. A year or two before he was arrested by the FBI, I found myself in a shouting match with Norman Seabrook, the head of the correction officers' union. Seabrook was berating a group of us on the health side about our interference in security decisions, namely, on where mentally ill inmates should be housed. As he spat venom at us, I started to make the point that ignoring our input often put his officers at risk when patients decompensated. He quickly shouted me down and said, "You shut the —— up; you go blow bubbles. Just go blow bubbles, that's all you do!" I was struck that in the midst of a fight about how differently we saw things, I didn't even understand the insult he was launching at me. I never figured out exactly what his reference was, but interactions like that reminded me that if we in the health service felt ignored and disrespected, imagine what it was like for our patients. The perspective of many jailers and their superiors at this time was that death and injury outcomes behind bars are the fault of the incarcerated. As a result, part of our responsibility in correctional health services was to point out how the jail system creates its own set of health risks for the people who pass through and to measure the uneven ways in which these risks are distributed across our patients based on gender, race, health status, and other variables.

Seabrook's influence was already clear to me from earlier incidents, including the beating of a patient named Jamal Lightfoot, who "eyeballed" a passing group of senior DOC leaders during a search. The DOC security chief, the top security official in the entire NYC jail system, allegedly told his team, "I want you to knock his f'in teeth in." This led to the inmate being cuffed, taken to an intake pen, and beaten until he had multiple facial fractures. This patient was later alleged either to have attacked DOC staff with a weapon or to have been hiding a weapon. The incident was so notorious that one of the senior staff involved put in his retirement papers within days. This senior security chief was close to Seabrook, and the *Daily News* ran a story in which Seabrook referenced this incident as justified use of force. The security chief was quickly asked to rescind his retirement by the commissioner of corrections, and he stayed on the job until his criminal indictment for this assault. He and a group of others involved in this assault would be convicted of multiple crimes, representing a dramatic departure from many years of acceptance of these acts.

Seabrook's power derived from an implicit threat that no other union could make: don't mess with us, or we can take over the jails. This may sound fantastic, but COBA had demonstrated their power once before. In 1990, a riot in one of the jails on Rikers Island led to the injury of several officers. The incident, as detailed in a State Commission of Corrections investigation, started when a violent altercation between a guard and an inmate in a single housing area spread to almost the entire jail. The riot occurred at a time when officers were understaffed, there were lapses in basic food and other services being delivered to inmates, and inmates had robbed and beaten a correction officer just days earlier. On the night of the violence, inmates in an area of the jail had fashioned both weapons and body armor from supplies they obtained in the jail. As an initial disturbance brought a riot team of correction officers into the housing area, they were quickly set upon, and three of them were slashed within minutes. When the officers in the Otis Bantum Correctional Center (OBCC) became overwhelmed, they sent a request for backup, resulting in 200 officers streaming across the bridge and from other jails, including many out of uniform and some apparently intoxicated.

With no central command in the jail, teams of correction officers began roving around, entering housing areas to battle with inmates. A total of 140 inmates were injured, with 95 requiring hospital treatment, and at least 36 were injured in dormitories where no disturbance took place. The New York State Commission of Correction (SCOC) report noted, "In one peaceable dormitory, 17 inmates were injured, including two with fractures, one compound finger fracture with partial amputation and one with head trauma with a ruptured eardrum. In suggesting that these injuries were accidental, the Department's incident report cannot be viewed as credible." The injuries to officers were mild and few by comparison, leading the SCOC to conclude that "the gross disparity between the nature and severity of correction officer and inmate injuries gives rise to profound doubts as to the degree of threat, use of weapons and extent of resistance."

I'd heard about this incident as lore, and it wasn't until I was in a heated meeting in 2014 that it came up again. I was there with my boss, Health Commissioner Mary Bassett, to meet with DOC Commissioner Ponte and his team. Somehow, COBA was alerted that we were meeting, and Norman Seabrook barged into the jail chapel where we were gathered. He strode right up to the pulpit and, in front of 30 or so senior DOC and health leadership staff, began lambasting Dr. Basset and the rest of us with insults and ridicule about our meddling in security matters like appropriate housing for the mentally ill. When it became clear that nobody in DOC was going to stop his profanity-laced tirade, we began to leave. In passing, a leader from COBA told a colleague from another agency, "Keep backing up health and we'll go back to 1990." This threat—to return to the OBCC takeover—is the basic one that COBA and every jail staff can make, for which there isn't much of an answer.

This was the power structure that we faced as we waded into the task of accurate injury reporting, but as the DOJ report came out in 2014 and press coverage of Rikers really blossomed, COBA also began to change their messaging in subtle but important ways. In 2015, Norman Seabrook began to say that reform wasn't the enemy, but that COBA and officers needed to be included in reform efforts. Further, he began to focus on the lack of resources and training for officers to deal with mentally ill patients. Seabrook's trial for corruption, which was tied to a wider case involving bribes in the government of NYC, resulted in a mistrial in 2017. COBA has continued to advocate for more officers (now with more than a 1:1 ratio to detainees) and solitary confinement, but with some tempering of their blind support of any use of force.

AN IMPORTANT PRODUCT from this work was our own understanding of the horrible impact that the culture of violence and neglect had on patients and staff alike. There's no doubt that the inmates who pass through these jails leave with trauma well beyond their physical injuries. Shortly after Mr. Hinton suffered his injuries, I went looking for another patient because a doctor said that he had witnessed the patient being beaten by officers in the jail clinic waiting area and that the patient had been dragged away without receiving care and had not been seen since. It took me a while to figure out which patient this might have been, and after failing to find him in any of the normal hiding spots in this jail, I went to another facility where "problematic" patients were often sent. I found him in a remote part of the second jail and heard him sobbing before I saw him in his cell. When I went to examine him, he lashed out wildly, still thinking he was going to be hit. It was clear that this patient had been injured well before I found him, and the officer who was working in that area quickly told me, "He was like that when they dropped him here."

The patients who experience these high levels of violence leave the jails with not only issues regarding trust but also hard lessons about the necessity of violence as a means of survival. The impact of this culture cuts both ways, however. On one night, I was in a jail to see a patient who had sustained multiple facial fractures during a use of force. He would ultimately tell me that he had been rear-cuffed and had his face smashed on a metal fixture as punishment for splashing an officer. When I got to the unit to see him, however, the only officer present to open his solitary cell was the same one who had been involved in the use of force the week before. The officer told me he wouldn't get the patient for me because of their history, and we waited for another officer to come. This started an awkward wait, with the two of us sitting side by side at a small table. We ended up talking, and when I asked about his time in this solitary unit, it became clear that he was dropped into this violent and chaotic setting right out of the DOC academy. Without guidance or training to the contrary, he used his size and strength to control the inmates who acted up. As he executed more and more uses of force, he received positive reinforcement for rough responses to inmates who acted up, and nothing in the way of an alternate approach. Before long, he developed a reputation for being able to handle the more difficult inmates. Talking to him, I was struck by the circumstances that molded him into this rough officer. Craig Haney, a colleague and mentor of mine, was part of the Stanford Prison Experiments, which involved dividing graduate students into two groups, one of prisoners and one of guards. In the experiment, as in a real jail or prison, the guards were given almost complete control over the prisoners, and within a few days the experiment was canceled because the grad students in the guard group were abusing the inmates. Imagine if that experiment had run for five or six years and the guards were given the impossible task of managing mentally ill inmates in solitary confinement. There are 10,000 correction officers in the NYC jail system, more than the number of inmates. While our primary focus regarding the health risks of incarceration is on the incarcerated, the effects on jail staff are also important to consider.

Ultimately, the only way to completely avoid violence and injuries in jail is to not be in jail. Every chapter in this book could end with this simple conclusion. But because every setting will tackle decarceration with different appetite and effectiveness, it's worth noting the real ways that injuries in jail can be reduced for the incarcerated. Most of the injuries in the NYC jails are intentional, violent injuries. Getting at the root causes of violence, especially in the chaos of jail, is an uphill trek. But one central observation from our injury work is that violence was used as a tool to control inmates. Although violence between correctional officer and inmate was the clearest evidence of this, we often received word of enforcement actions where officers directed one set of inmates to attack another. Relying on one group of inmates to control another is almost universal in jails and prisons, but when this includes beatings or extortion, the rules of the institution become replaced with a more Machiavellian code. In 2008, 18-year-old Chris Robinson was killed when correction officers allowed one group of inmates to enter his cell and beat him to death. This death revealed widespread violence in that jail, including the allegations that correction officers were running fight clubs among inmates.[11] These conditions were not confined to one jail, and the use of violence as a tool of control continued to be supported for several more years. But like in other settings where abuse is rationalized as a tool of control, it's almost never used in the judicious or even-handed manner that the abusers would like you to believe. One of the 129 patients in the use-of-force report who made an impression on me was a middle-aged man who spoke up because officers were taking muffins meant for the inmates.

He told me that after he filed a complaint about the muffins, officers and a captain showed up to his housing area and pulled him out into the hallway, where they berated him for making the complaint and then beat him with their fists and struck him in the face with a radio. He told me that as he lay injured with serious facial and head injuries, the officers then stopped two passing inmates and told them that they would be written up as being in a fight with this man, but that they would escape any real punishment if they went along with the story.

Because violence was used as a tool of control in a setting that requires control, the key to reducing the bad uses of force is to give officers another, more effective and humane tool. In the past year, DOC and health staff have begun rolling out an approach that is clearly linked to violence reduction during use of force: the CIT.[12] In community policing, use of CITs has been standard for more than a decade, with the goal of training police officers to work in teams with mental health professionals to de-escalate situations that involve emotionally disturbed people. I know the benefits of crisis intervention training firsthand, having worked with DOC officers to de-escalate many conflicts with our patients. One of my favorite patients ever, a brash and outspoken woman, once lay down on the floor of a jail clinic and screamed that she wouldn't move until someone listened to her. This patient was so feared and reviled by the security service that her movements and interactions with staff were always captured on video camera, to protect against future lawsuits. When I arrived in the jail clinic, she was sitting on the floor surrounded by a confused array of security and health staff. I plopped down next to her on the floor, and after 10 minutes of listening to her, she and I got a sense of what she was most upset about, and we came up with a plan for how to address some of her concerns. She and I still cross paths at public events about Rikers, and the short time we spent on the floor made it possible for us to have real conversations later on, even when I wasn't in a position to address all the problems she would raise.

Because ours was the first jail system to adopt crisis intervention training, we sent a team of health and security staff for CIT training at the Barbara Schneider Foundation in Minnesota.[13] This team was led by DOC deputy warden John Gallagher and our own deputy director of mental health, Anthony Waters. Deputy Gallagher had worked with me and many others to de-escalate volatile incidents with patients. The team returned to Rikers, developed its own 40-hour program, including training scenarios with mock patients, and set about training as many health and security staff as possible. Our early data indicate that the program is helping to dramatically reduce use of force in the buildings where it's being used. The team activations occur much like a probe team would be activated. Officers notify central command of a problem requiring assistance. The senior security officer then considers whether the CIT of three or four security and health staff could respond. If so, the team gathers some quick information about the patient and walks to the area with the goal of defusing the situation. Imagine the difference in outcomes in responding to angry or agitated people when a CIT can replace the process of assembling 10 officers who don riot gear and march in lockstep down the hall beating batons to shields. Maybe the best benefit of the CIT is found outside these official team activations. The officers who go through the program start to implement their skills in little ways many times each week, from getting patients to go to court to settling small disputes in housing areas that are ready to escalate to a fight. In one of the jails where CITs have been rolled out with great success, the warden makes announcements congratulating officers for de-escalation, something almost unimaginable a few years ago.

When considering Mr. Hinton's case and the injury data we compiled, there are two responses that we've received from skeptics. First, some think that if violent inmates were out on the street, they would also be getting injured there. It's true that poor and underserved communities, from which most incarcerated people come, have higher injury rates, sometimes as high as 250 or 300 injuries per 1,000 person-years. This would mean that for every three or four years of life lived in these settings, one could expect a single injury. But the data from the jails, where most people were being held before their trials and for nonviolent offenses, revealed a horrifying contrast. The rate of injury that we found in the jails in our original analysis was many times higher, 736 per 1,000 person-years.

The other comment we sometimes receive is that because we were the first jail to report this type of analysis, what was to say that the reported number of injuries was too high? Maybe this is just how jails are. It's a perverse but vexing response. I think that the rates of injury in the NYC jails are likely higher than in many other settings, but the DOJ should be mandating standardized injury reporting from every jail and prison for comparison, so we all can know the truth. This would not only alert parties outside the walls to problems within but also insulate some more progressive settings when a single bad outcome leads to litigation. Being able to say that a facility is at or better than the national average for an important outcome would help many cities and counties defending lawsuits. Nonetheless, being injured or subject to violence is a concern for every incarcerated person. The loss of autonomy and security, combined with the natural tendency for inmates and security staff alike to abuse their power over the more vulnerable around them, renders these settings inherently violent. It's likely true that the problems of violence in the NYC jail system are worse than in some other settings. But we don't really know what happens in most other settings, largely because the type of data we gathered either doesn't exist elsewhere or won't ever see the light of day.

Rikers mirrored the rest of the nation's jails in this respect until a horrible outcome prompted a smarter response. This type of surveillance program is exactly what Commissioner Freiden told us to build after Christopher Robinson's death, and Freiden's successors, Commissioners Farley and Bassett, supported my team in implementing the plan despite ample resistance from security staff and other city officials. By designing our EMR to collect data about inmates' injuries, their environment, and their personal profiles, all as structured variables, we were able to quickly assemble large-scale reports that were helpful to the DOJ and the press once obtained through freedom of information requests. Without this external pressure, the city would not have been forced toward reform. While violence remains high overall, one of the clear recent improvements in the NYC jail system is a decrease in serious injuries during uses of force. This improvement has been one of the few bright spots in the jails, and even if the culture of violence reasserts itself, the reliance on and demand for data on these outcomes won't easily be undone.

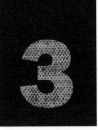

Solitary Confinement

WALKING DOWN THE LONG HALLWAY to the solitary unit where he would die, Jason Echevarria passed two messages painted across the ceiling beams: "Maintain self-respect" and "Improve the moment." Mr. Echevarria died several weeks later, and it was one of the longest and most painful deaths I have investigated in any jail. The initial act that set these events in motion reveals the terrible health consequences of solitary confinement, just as damaging as the abuse hours later that led to Mr. Echevarria's death. In an effort to escape the stress of solitary confinement, Mr. Echevarria swallowed a packet of industrial soap and then told correctional officers that he needed medical attention. Passing medical staff confirmed that he was vomiting and required medical attention, but the response of Department of Correction staff and their supervisor was to keep Mr. Echevarria in his cell overnight, intermittently taunting and ignoring him as he vomited blood, bile, and lye, screamed for help, and ultimately died with an eroded esophagus. While most of the focus on Mr. Echevarria's case was rightly centered on the role of DOC staff in causing his death, an equal measure of horror should be reserved for the thought that Mr. Echevarria and hundreds of thousands of other people routinely experience solitary confinement and some of them prefer harming or even killing themselves to continued exposure to these settings.

Solitary confinement is the practice of placing the incarcerated into a small cell alone for 23 or 24 hours a day. This practice represents one of the most dramatic health risks of incarceration, and the gruesome and preventable death of Mr. Echevarria should etch the failures of this approach into our consciousness. Mr. Echevarria was just 25 when he died after swallowing a packet known in the New York City jails as a "soap ball" in 2012.[1] He did this to escape solitary confinement, where he was being held as punishment, and under normal circumstances, he would have succeeded. Because officers know that these soap balls are toxic, Mr. Echevarria's actions should have resulted in him being taken out of his cell for prompt medical evaluation. Unfortunately, Mr. Echevarria was known to DOC staff as a "bing beater," someone who correctional staff (and some health staff) thought was just trying to get out of his punishment. His death in solitary confinement focused our attention on the health risks of this practice, even among people who were not judged to be the most seriously ill. Thousands of patients each year were being punished for even minor jail offenses with solitary confinement, and their behavioral problems seemed to get worse inside "the box," including harm to themselves. When we raised these observations with key policy makers, we were met with a request for data—something more compelling than the opinion of doctors about their patients.

The circumstances of Mr. Echevarria's death are as horrifying as one will find inside a jail anywhere. On the eve of his death, Mr. Echevarria was being held in the violent Mental Health Assessment Unit for Infracted Inmates, the special solitary confinement unit for people with mental illness who disobeyed jail rules. In theory, the MHAUII was a regular solitary confinement unit (23 or 24 hours per day locked in a cell) with extra mental health staff present to check on patients. In practice, it was the most violent unit in the jail system, with patients taking extreme measures to gain attention and often making desperate attempts to get themselves removed. The extra mental health staff in these units were essentially bystanders to this brutality, sometimes removing patients to the hospital or other mental health settings. When Mr. Echevarria entered solitary, the NYC jail system's dependence on solitary was very high, with over 7 percent of adults and 25 percent of adolescents going into "the box." Contrary to most developed nations, solitary confinement is a significant feature of American correctional practice. Placing incarcerated individuals alone in a cell for extended periods of time was first routinized in Philadelphia in 1829 when Quakers worked to reform a violent and abusive penitentiary system.[2] In that model, people were locked in stone cells alone with a bible, with the goal being to promote closeness to God and introspection about past acts. The result of this practice was often suicide, loss of sanity, or decreased social functioning. After Charles Dickens toured the facility in 1842, he wrote,

> I believe that very few men are capable of estimating the immense amount
> of torture and agony which this dreadful punishment, prolonged for years,
> inflicts upon the sufferers. . . . I hold this slow and daily tampering with
> the mysteries of the brain to be immeasurably worse than any torture of
> the body; and because its ghastly signs and tokens are not so palpable to
> the eye and sense of touch as scars upon the flesh; because its wounds are
> not upon the surface, and it extorts few cries that human ears can hear;
> therefore the more I denounce it, as a secret punishment which slum-
> bering humanity is not roused up to stay.[3]

Later that century, the US Supreme Court took a similar view of the practice, when Justice Miller (also a physician) observed of the Philadelphia system that "a considerable number of the prisoners fell, after even a short confinement, into a semi-fatuous condition, from which it was next to impossible to arouse them, and others became violently insane; others still, committed suicide; while those who stood the ordeal better were not generally reformed, and in most cases did not recover sufficient mental activity to be of any subsequent service to the community."[4]

Owing to the lack of reformative success with this method, as well as the negative ruling of the US Supreme Court, the practice of solitary confinement fell out of practice for almost a century. Some correctional systems would maintain a small number of cells for solitary confinement to punish the most egregious offenses inside their walls, including "The Hole" or D Block at Alcatraz in the early 1900s.

Modern reliance on solitary confinement grew out of desperation when two correctional officers were killed by inmates on the same day at the US Penitentiary in Marion in 1982. The warden of that facility put the entire prison on "permanent lockdown," eliminating all educational, work, and other programs. This reaction to violent deaths of security staff became the blueprint for the Pelican Bay State Prison in 1989, an entire jail purposely built for solitary confinement, with no need for any congregate spaces such as classrooms, commissary, cafeterias, or other settings of social interaction. After Pelican Bay, the first of the "supermax" facilities, this model was repeated many times over. By 1990, approximately 30 states were operating these types of facilities, and by 2005, 40 states were in the supermax business.[5]

Although prisoners' rights advocates and mental health professionals raised alarm over the growth of solitary confinement during this period, the discussion was almost entirely about prisons. Two of the leading voices in this area have been Drs. Craig Haney and Terry Kupers.[6] Together, these and other academic mental health researchers have provided expert testimony and research on the topic of solitary confinement, mostly in prison systems. Because of the chaos and short stays that characterized jails, little information is available to outsiders about solitary confinement or health outcomes of people held there. In addition, while prisons tended to use solitary confinement for administrative segregation (a preventive form of separation, based on overall dangerousness), jails often rely on solitary confinement for punitive reasons, such as for violation of jail rules. The infraction process inside jails represents an arbitrary and hidden system of adjudication and punishment for the incarcerated. People charged with violating jail rules can face financial fines, loss of visitation and other privileges, and placement in solitary confinement. In addition, throughout this secretive infraction practice, people have no rights to representation or other basic aspects of fair review.

DURING THE DAYS WHEN the MHAUII was in operation, we routinely observed that people with mental health problems would enter jail and have trouble coping with the arbitrary and complex set of rules they were expected to follow. Then, when they did come into conflict with the rules, they were placed in settings with even tighter control, less autonomy, and more arbitrariness. Once inside the MHAUII or another solitary facility, patients would rack up many more infractions, to the point of absurdity. Unfortunately, there are real consequences for these infractions. One patient in the MHAUII attempted suicide by breaking off a sprinkler head to use in slashing his wrist. Some weeks after the incident, when the patient was recovering in the hospital, staff informed me that the patient had received a new infraction, plus a new criminal charge for destruction of government property, as well as a fine for the sprinkler repair. Our staff told DOC to remove the patient from solitary to receive treatment, but when I expressed shock at the patient being charged and fined for attempting to harm himself because of the setting he had been placed in, the response I received was basically, "This is expensive equipment."

Punishing men and women for the anguish and pain *caused* by solitary confinement is at the heart of Mr. Echevarria's tragedy. On the night in question, Mr. Echevarria and other patients in this solitary unit found themselves in a familiar but insane circumstance. One of the patients in the upper level of cells had blocked his toilet, leading his and other toilets to back up and spill raw sewage across the floor and into adjacent cells and those on the bottom tier. I have been on these units when sewage-filled water pours out of one cell and spreads across the entire unit, and the smell is overpowering. Often the sewage and water mix with food trays laying on the floor, and the stench is quickly made worse by the presence of insects, mice, and other vermin. Also, the routine nature of these floods meant that DOC plumbers were frequently running between these units, and it was often a day or two before a unit was cleaned. Jail wardens and other managers would often decide to "let them stew," a line of reasoning that pervades corrections and is based on the idea that individuals who engage in bad acts will bring consequences for the entire unit. But for Mr. Echevarria and the others, officers decided to toss "soap balls" into their cells. These soap balls are about the size of those used in laundry machines, but much stronger. In fact, these industrial cleaners were so concentrated that they were designed to be dissolved into five-gallon mop buckets. But on Mr. Echevarria's unit, the security staff gave them to individual inmates as a means to clean their own cells. The lack of wisdom in having inmates slop raw sewage out of their cells notwithstanding, Mr. Echevarria quickly seized on the opportunity and ingested one or more of the soap balls. This act of self-harm was not uncommon among people who wanted to escape the rigors or chaos of the MHAUII or other solitary units. Mr. Echevarria quickly told a passing health staffer what he had done, who in turn informed security staff of the incident and that Mr. Echevarria needed quick medical evaluation, with risk of death if he wasn't checked out. According to press reports and the criminal complaints from the case, not only did security staff fail to remove Mr. Echevarria from his cell, but a supervisor came to the area and told officers not to bother him, stating that they should call him back "when they had a body." Mr. Echevarria had already started to vomit and was yelling for help. As the hours passed by, the security officers continued to look into Mr. Echevarria's cell, he continued to vomit and yell for help, and other inmates started to yell for him to be removed. Sometime late in the evening, there was an unexplained power outage, causing the cameras on the unit to stop functioning, so events after midnight are not recorded. Mr. Hinton, who had his neck and facial bones broken on this same unit, also had an unexplained gap in camera coverage. Accounts from the other inmates on the unit are harrowing. Mr. Echevarria was screaming and pleading for help. Security staff taunted him. The lights were out, and raw sewage coated the cells. As some point, Mr. Echevarria's cries stopped. When the lights and video cameras came back on, Jason Echevarria was dead in his cell. I've been back on this unit many times and thought about what these hours were like for Mr. Echevarria and the others on the unit. The only historical comparison that I can make is the slave ships that transported kidnapped Africans across the Atlantic. The brutality, isolation, widespread misery, and mocking and indifference as someone slowly dies seem like the type of hellish circumstances that must have been encountered by Africans chained below decks for months in slave ships.

At Mr. Echevarria's autopsy, the medical examiner found extensive erosion and burning along his esophagus, along with aspiration of vomit into his lungs. His death was painful and prolonged. Local prosecutors decided not to pursue any criminal charges against the security staff in this case; however, almost two years after his death, the US attorney took up the case and secured a conviction against the DOC supervisor and a five-year prison sentence.

There is no doubt that the refusal to remove Mr. Echevarria from his cell resulted in his death. The investigation into his ingestion of the soap balls and the prosecution of the DOC captain were crucial to addressing the most immediate concerns in this case. But any discussion with health or security staff in the MHAUII would reveal that this type of occurrence was common; only the death was rare. Patients often harmed themselves to get out of solitary, and their acts of self-harm were often viewed as contrived and malingering. This view would put health staff in the impossible position of trying to judge whether a person's actions reflected mental illness or a desire to be somewhere else. In addition, the high levels of violence in the MHAUII led staff and patients alike to resort to extreme methods of interaction, such as patients splashing staff with urine or feces and staff beating patients after they had been restrained. Because solitary units like the MHAUII are created for punishment, health staff are not only asked to conduct am impossible clinical assessment; they're asked to do it in a violent and chaotic setting. The outcome of this ridiculous approach is best predicted by the power dynamic of the setting: health staff will provide assessments that meet the demands of the security staff if they rely on those same staff for their safety and well-being. As we reviewed this case internally, we concluded that the setting of the MHAUII and the practice of solitary confinement were key contributors to Mr. Echevarria's death. When we engaged with key decision makers on this issue, advocating for elimination of the MHAUII, we were again asked for data to prove our point.

At the time of Mr. Echevarria's death, there were not any large-scale analyses of health outcomes associated with solitary confinement in jails. Even the analyses available from prisons revealed a slight increase in rate of suicide and not much else. The rest of the literature amounted to personal opinion and small cohort analyses, relatively weak in terms of level of evidence. Equally important, jails are vastly different from prisons. The chaos of jails results in higher rates of violence and less certainty about health and security labels. In addition, because people spend shorter and less predictable amounts of time in jail, the profile of long-term solitary confinement (e.g., Pelican Bay) is less relevant. As we mobilized our data team to analyze the health impact of solitary confinement in our setting, the clinical observations in Mr. Echevarria's case resonated. He and other patients would do horrible things to themselves to escape or avoid solitary. The harm was real; the issue of what was in their hearts was an academic one. Patients still became gravely ill (or died) as a result of this self-harm. By the time Mr. Echevarria died, we had already noticed a dramatic increase in the rate of self-harm, and our analysis of these acts would reveal a clear association with solitary confinement. We leveraged our electronic medical record to analyze about 225,000 jail admissions over a three-year period.[7] Among the most significant findings of this analysis, only 7 percent of people in jail ever went into solitary, but more than half of all the self-harm cases were found in this small group. To look at it another way, people going into solitary are 6.9 times more likely to hurt themselves. Other predictors of self-harm were serious mental illness and being an adolescent. In addition, when we looked at potentially fatal cases of self-harm, solitary confinement and serious mental illness were still highly predictive factors. Equally shocking, we found that for every 100 acts of self-harm, there were 36 transfers to higher levels of care (on-island urgent care or local emergency room), 10 hospital admissions, 3,760 hours of correction officer escort time (usually working overtime), and 450 excess clinical encounters in the jails. This reliance on overtime staff raised the specter of a system that was not just harmful but also expensive. Every time a person being held in solitary was transported to the Rikers emergency center or to a local hospital, at least two officers would "escort" the detainee. For most serious injuries, the transfer to Bellevue or another hospital could take 12–24 hours even if the treatment was relatively uncomplicated. These runs could easily consume six or eight officer shifts, almost all of which were done by officers working overtime because of the unpredictable nature of the time required. In addition, anyone who has been in an emergency room when an arrestee or prisoner arrives with escort officers can understand how disruptive this process is for the emergency department. Thousands of these transfers were occurring every year, driven by the jail system's addiction to solitary confinement. Taken together, these data helped us display the evidence of harms to individuals and larger systems that were caused by solitary confinement.

At the local level, the gruesome and preventable death of Mr. Echevarria and our data analysis about self-harm helped us to prevail in eliminating the MHAUII and the practice of using solitary confinement for seriously mentally ill people in jail.[8] Many other forces were already in play on this issue. Before Mr. Echevarria's death, there had been increasing focus on the health problems associated with solitary confinement for several years among jail reform advocates, and the violence in the MHAUII was attracting scrutiny from the jail oversight body, the NYC Board of Correction, and litigators. We had shared data on injuries for adult and adolescent patients in the MHAUII with the US Department of Justice, which was preparing a civil rights suit against NYC DOC, and their investigations led them to visit the MHAUII and interview patients there.[9] In addition, we had written a brief to our supervisors shortly before Mr. Echevarria's death in response to DOC asking for *expansion* of the MHAUII. In this brief, we gave our medical opinion that the MHAUII and solitary confinement in general were harmful for our patients and that we should eliminate this practice for our patients with mental illness and adolescents and severely limit it for all others.

While this memo didn't result in policy changes, it did galvanize all of us who signed it, including almost all of the senior leadership in correctional health, as well as some at Bellevue Hospital. It also served notice that the city's doctors viewed a common practice of the city as harmful to patients. By the time we completed our self-harm analysis, the discussion was shifting from DOC wanting more solitary for the mentally ill to completely eliminating the practice. We'd structured our analysis to find the variables most associated with self-harm, and since serious mental illness and being adolescent were the two variables most predictive of self-harm, we were able to make an evidence-based argument to exclude these groups from solitary. It's important to keep in mind that our analysis identified a serious risk of self-harm for all persons who ever passed into solitary, so while these improvements were welcome, they were (and remain) incomplete, since solitary persists.

Having attained prohibition from entering solitary confinement for persons with serious mental illness and adolescents, we then worked to design and fund new models of care. The first step was the creation of a special treatment unit for patients with serious mental illness who run afoul of jail rules. This unit, called the Clinical Alternative to Punitive Segregation (CAPS) unit, would be a significant step forward for the patients who passed through it, but the drive to really reduce the practice of solitary confinement would take another two to three years and more intervention by oversight bodies. The CAPS unit was based on clinical engagement instead of punishment, and entry and exit were directed by clinical staff, not security managers. On these units, patients had a broad array of programs available to them, including group and individual therapy, art therapy, and other activities. In addition, these units had a rich allotment of staff, including mental health aides who could spend their entire shift interacting with patients and noting who was faring poorly before an incident occurred.

OUTSIDE NYC, THE DATA we had gathered quickly became part of the discussion about the safety and wisdom of solitary confinement. The self-harm paper received some national press coverage when we published it in

2014 and was awarded the Paper of the Year by the *American Journal of Public Health*. That acclaim helped get the data into the hands of others considering the issue of solitary confinement.[10] We began to see our data reflected in lawsuits around the country challenging the appropriateness of solitary confinement, as well as in reports on the topic by the United Nations and the US Civil Rights Commission.[11] At the same time, a new analysis from Texas addressed a basic but forgotten question: does solitary work? Dr. Robert Morris, a criminologist at the University of Texas at Dallas, analyzed data from over 3,000 state prisoners across 70 prisons.[12] He found that inmates who had committed an initial violent offense were no less likely to commit a second violent act if they were punished with solitary confinement, and the time between a first and second violent act was not changed by punishment with solitary confinement. This study seems to be the first to specifically examine the question of solitary's effectiveness and added to the weight of concerns about solitary confinement. Maybe the most significant role for these data on the national scene came in 2015, when the issue of solitary confinement returned to the US Supreme Court. In a 2015 death penalty case that didn't appear to overtly involve solitary confinement, Justice Kennedy wrote, "In a case that presented the issue, the judiciary may be required to determine whether workable alternative systems for long-term confinement exist, and, if so, whether a correctional system should be required to adopt them."[13] Justice Kennedy cited our self-harm data in his opinion, and his striking commentary was widely interpreted as an invitation to review the broad matter of solitary confinement in the coming sessions of the Supreme Court. The death of Jason Echeverria did not start or end the discussion about solitary confinement. Neither did our analysis of self-harm. But the horror of Mr. Echeverria's death and the clarity of our data both helped to shine a spotlight on this issue at an important time in NYC.

On the opening day of the pure mental health unit that replaced the MHAUII, I pointed out to newly hired staff the cell where Mr. Echeverria died. They had a hard time conceiving of how he was allowed to die and focused on the failures of individuals involved in his case. But the lessons of the MHAUII are many, and among them is that we cannot create restrictive and brutal settings and then be surprised when staff and patients alike respond poorly. Mr. Echeverria and the other 244,698 jail admissions included in our analysis reveal that the risks imparted by the jail environment are considerable, for anyone, and that some groups face higher risks than others. The lack of evidence behind solitary confinement as an effective tool in jails, combined with the costly health consequences of these settings, should push us to eliminate it as a form of jail punishment.

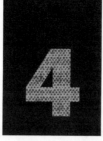

Serious Mental Illness in Jail

T**HE DEATH OF** B**RADLEY** B**ALLARD** at Rikers reveals how dangerous jail can be for mentally ill patients. While the medical examiner identified sepsis and diabetes as causes of death for Mr. Ballard, the real reason he died is that the jail system was completely unable to manage his needs. When Mr. Ballard exhibited routine signs of his mental illness, the system responded with a fatal mix of abuse and neglect. Mr. Ballard was 39 when he was arrested in Houston, Texas, for exposing himself to a bus driver. He was on parole from a prior incarceration in New York, and since he was in Texas without having notified his parole officer, he was extradited to New York and taken directly to Rikers. Once there, his conflicts with other patients and correctional staff led to him being diagnosed with serious mental illness. But like many other before him, Mr. Ballard received a confused patchwork of punishment and treatment while incarcerated. Ultimately, he repeated the same behaviors inside jail that led to his arrest in Houston, and the response of security staff was to lock him in a cell for a week, against all policies of his mental health unit. During this time, health staff who went to his unit did not realize that Mr. Ballard had been locked away with his water turned off, and they also failed to check on his worsening condition. Unknown to everyone, on the day he was locked into his cell, Mr. Ballard had tied a ligature around his genitals, leading to a massive tissue necrosis and, ultimately, a fatal infection. Because of the reporting done by the Associated Press and the *New York Times* on this and other cases, city officials took substantial steps to give us in correctional health and security staff the resources needed to ensure that this type of tragedy was not repeated. We built new therapeutic mental health units modeled after inpatient psychiatric centers, with teams of health and security staff who worked together every day caring for the same patients, and with many more staff and programs for patients. These units meet the obligation we have to patients like Mr. Ballard, but their cost and complexity should cause us all to reconsider the wisdom of jail as a place for people with serious mental illness. Moreover, some of the basic failings in Mr. Bradley's case were never addressed; I left Rikers just as concerned about patients languishing for days in cells as I was when I started. The lack of meaningful improvements to the tracking and accountability for custody management lies at the core of Riker's unresolved issues. On the clinical side, we failed Mr. Ballard, and now having built the type of clinical unit that he needed, it seems unlikely that most settings will have the resources or independence to do the same.

Bradley Ballard's journey to Rikers began on a public bus in Houston in the summer of 2013.[1] Mr. Ballard's arrest and transfer to Rikers occurred in June, and he would die there three months later. Mr. Ballard was initially placed in a general population housing area, but behavioral problems in the jail led him to be transferred to the inpatient psychiatric ward at Bellevue Hospital, where he received high-level care for his serious mental illness. He spent 38 days at Bellevue before being sent back to Rikers, where he was placed in a "mental observation" unit. At the time, we had about 25 such units, and they were dedicated to patients with mental health issues who needed more support and care than was available in general population housing areas. The reality of these units was varied; some of them had health and correctional staff who worked the same unit every day and worked as a team to find patients who needed help with medication compliance, individual or group therapy, or hospital transfer. But in many of these settings, the health staff in place only visited the unit for a few minutes a day, and the security staff rotated through with little training, resources, or interest in managing the unit. As a result of not having a team of health and security staff who worked on many of these units, there was little incentive to find patients who were faring poorly, and a larger incentive to just ignore problems until the end of a shift, leaving the issue for someone else. In addition, none of these units had the critical psychiatric technicians or mental health aides that are a staple of inpatient psychiatric hospitals. These staff have less training than psychologists or social workers, but they perform essential functions in helping patients get to and from programs, working to resolve small disputes that can quickly escalate, and serving as a constant set of eyes and ears to detect patients who are becoming sicker. To make matters worse, most of these units were physically designed for punishment, with little open space for programs or group activities and such decrepit walls, floors, and ceilings that is was easy to fashion weapons from almost any surface. The jail with the greatest number of these mental observation units is the Anna M. Kross Center, the largest in the jail system. Of the 2,200 people held in this jail, about 400 are in mental observation units. Although the health services team is responsible for admitting and discharging patients from these units, another glaring weakness in this system is that if a patient like Mr. Ballard has a behavioral problem, the security staff could just move him from one mental observation unit to another, without notifying health staff. The antiquated system used by the Department of Correction to track the location of inmates could take days to show a new location, leaving mental health, pharmacy, and other staff completely unaware of a patient's whereabouts. This same system was still in place and failing in the same manner when I left Rikers in 2017. As a result of these shortcomings, patients like Mr. Ballard were often difficult for health staff to find, despite having a modern electronic medical record and medical, nursing, and pharmacy staff who were ready to give out medications.

THE LACK OF TIMELY INFORMATION about patients has been at the heart of numerous preventable deaths in our system. In 2012, Gregory Gionatta, a 41-year-old man with bipolar disease, was brought to Rikers with a note from a physician stating that he was suicidal. This paper was noted by correctional officers before he entered the jail, but it didn't prompt an immediate suicide watch or any sort of system-wide alert to all the staff members who would interact with him.[2] Tragically, like thousands of other pieces of paper that make their way into the jails every month, this critical letter wasn't produced to medical staff until after he hanged himself in the bathroom of the jail intake. In 2013, 35-year-old Horsone Moore hanged himself in the same jail's intake area after several observed suicide attempts. One year later, after mental health staff saw patient Fabian Cruz, they initiated a suicide watch and ordered a transfer to a mental health unit, but he was returned to his housing area in error, where he committed suicide.[3] Although the New York City jail system has a rate of suicide that's lower than the national average, these tragedies reflect the poor linkage in critical information systems between health and security services. For Mr. Ballard and others, the health consequences of the breakdown of this interface between paper and electronic processes were dire. When patients like Mr. Ballard were moved from one spot to another without any new information being entered into the security system, our EMR (and staff) would continue to assume he was in the first location. This uncertainty about location creates the need for medical, mental health, pharmacy, and nursing staff to roam the halls of the jails every day physically looking for their patients. The impact of flying blind goes well beyond the mental health service and suicide risk.

In 2013, a patient named Ronaldo Perez died of seizures while locked in solitary confinement. This 36-year-old man was very vocal about needing his anti-seizure medications, and at his original facility he had been placed on a special list to ensure directly observed therapy (DOT) so that staff would know that his medications had been taken. Unbeknownst to health staff, he was transferred from one jail to another and placed in solitary confinement over a weekend. According to other inmates in this solitary unit, he repeatedly asked correctional officers to bring him to the clinic for his medication, but his pleas were ignored for days, and he died of seizures on that unit.[4] The actions of the officers notwithstanding, the inability of health staff to locate him was a major factor in his death.

The inability to find patients like Mr. Ballard was made worse by the cultural debate about whether patients with serious mental illness deserve treatment or punishment. For the 38 days he was in the care of the forensic ward at Bellevue, Mr. Ballard received daily care from a team that had the resources and autonomy to improve his condition. The Bellevue Prison Ward is a national model, with about 100 beds dedicated to medical and mental health care of patients too sick for the jails. The 19th floor of the hospital is set up with many of the same features of a jail, including the bubble, sally port, and correctional officers. But the unit is in a hospital, so the dominant priority is care. Patients are seen when the health staff want to see them, medications are readily accessible, and when emergencies occur, other hospital staff can come to assist. Dr. Budd Heyman runs the medical side of the floor and has established a setting where our patients receive the best possible care when they become too ill for our infirmary. Dr. Elizabeth Ford was the head of the forensic (mental health) wings when Mr. Ballard was there, and she achieved a critical transformation in that unit by working with her staff and the correctional officers to reduce uses of force by officers and increase the engagement of patients in their own care. Her staff even developed a drama program for patients, which was an incredible motivator to participate in treatment because everyone wanted to be part of the play on the floor. Dr. Ford's leadership on the Bellevue forensic unit led me to recruit her to lead our own psychiatric service in the jail in 2015, and she recently published her own book detailing her experiences leading the Bellevue forensic service. Her observations about the intersection between humanity and psychiatric care for patients in the Bellevue Prison Ward bring into high relief what is lacking in most correctional health settings.[5]

For Mr. Ballard, this high level of care would be fractured when he returned to Rikers. This cycle is painfully common for patients with schizophrenia, bipolar disease, and other forms of serious mental illness, especially those who are poor. While being cared for in a hospital, they usually receive psychiatric care that correctly identifies their problems and delivers medications and other care to pull them back from the brink of being psychotic or actively suicidal. Once stable, however, they are sent back to jail, where the violence, chaos, and lack of mental health resources essentially cause them to decompensate again.

When Mr. Ballard returned to jail from Bellevue, his problems escalated. He was transferred to a new mental health unit after a fight. By this time, Mr. Ballard was clearly exhibiting worsening signs of serious mental illness, and review of his chart would also reveal numerous missed medical and medication appointments. Once in his new housing area, Mr. Ballard made a lewd gesture toward a correction officer. In response, he was locked in his cell, in violation of the entire idea of mental observation units. By design, these units were set up not only to provide care but also to "observe" patients so that staff could transfer them to the hospital when they decompensated. For a patient like Mr. Ballard, suffering from schizophrenia, decompensation may include very noticeable symptoms such as auditory or visual hallucinations, paranoia, impaired judgment, and conflict. Other symptoms can be less obvious, like staring off into space or going long periods of time with-out speaking or interacting with others. Patients on this unit were supposed to receive their regularly scheduled mental health and medical visits, but there was also supposed to be something called "rounding" that involved a social worker visiting the housing area daily to make sure nobody was de-compensating. On the day of his incident with the correctional officer, Mr. Ballard was locked in his cell, and when he flooded his toilet out of protest, his water was shut off. Over the next seven days, he would remain in that cell, never coming out for any mental health or medical encounter or for his multiple medications. Although missing an appointment or medica-tion raises concerns among health staff, only about half of all patients were being brought to our health clinics for their scheduled encounters during this time, so health staff faced an impossible task of triage every day, strug-gling to find the missed appointments and medications that were most seri-ous. However, the scant health staff who visited this unit while Mr. Ballard was there failed to perform their basic assessments of his status or notice that his water was cut off. Over the next seven days, officers of increasing rank would stop and look into Mr. Ballard's cell with increasing frequency. None of them let him out. None ordered his water turned on. This isola-tion from care hastened Mr. Ballard's deterioration from his schizophrenia as well as infection. The sewage stench and other odors were so strong that correctional officers would spray air freshener into Mr. Ballard's cell, and the inmate worker who passed out food trays was seen on video covering his face when he passed Mr. Ballard's cell. This pattern is sadly familiar. In jail, when there is a general sense of a patient getting worse, it often results in increasing surveillance but no meaningful intervention. By day 7, Mr. Ballard was apparently not moving much, and a medical emergency was called. When the medical team arrived, they found Mr. Ballard slumped on the floor, covered in feces, with a stench so strong that they had difficulty entering the cell. Mr. Ballard went into cardiac arrest soon thereafter, and by the time he arrived at Elmhurst Hospital, he had been declared dead.

Inside the jails, Mr. Ballard's death was viewed as horrific and prevent-able, but it was clearly a product of widespread dysfunction. We found that staff and leadership working for the health staffing company, Corizon, had failed at basic responsibilities like conducting daily rounds of Mr. Ballard's unit. But those failures were facilitated because of their own chronic staffing shortages, security staff neglecting to bring patients to the medical clinic, and health staff not knowing where patients were housed. Most glaringly, responding to behavioral problems in a mental health unit by locking someone in a cell and turning off their water was beyond the pale of reasonable behavior. This feature of Mr. Ballard's death evokes the tragedy of Mr. Ramirez, who was beaten to death by correctional staff. Mr. Ramirez was identified as needing special care and housing for his risk of going into alcohol withdrawal, but when he did just that, he was beaten to death. The New York State Commission on Corrections, a state oversight body, agreed with our assessment of the pervasive failings in Mr. Ballard's case. They concluded that the mental health unit had been effectively turned into a solitary confinement area despite our intentions.

The death of Bradley Ballard was a horrible outcome of a national shift in how we approach mental illness. Several decades ago, someone with a serious mental illness was more likely to be cared for in a hospital than jail or prison. In 1960, the United States could house 550,000 people in mental health hospitals. But out of concern that institutionalizing people with mental illness was a violation of their rights, most patients were released to be cared for in the community. This transition wouldn't have been so catastrophic if there had been a matching commitment to develop community (outpatient) mental health resources, with more supportive housing linked to outpatient care. By 2011, nearly all mental health institutions had been closed, and today space remains for just 43,000 people.[6] Since that time, the number of prison and jail beds has gone from about 300,000 to 2.3 million. Consequently, the multiple policy misadventures of the war on drugs and dismantling of the nation's mental health service have transformed jails and prisons into the de facto mental health service for the poor and especially for minorities. And now, when someone with serious mental illness acts violent or lewd, there is a very good chance that they'll end up in a jail, rather than in a mental health facility. In the nine years I worked at Rikers, the proportion of inmates who were in the mental health service rose from about one-third to about one-half. More alarmingly, the percentage of people with serious mental illness, like Mr. Ballard, climbed steadily from about 5 percent of the daily census to 11 percent. All of this occurred against the backdrop of great success in *lowering* the jail population of NYC. Analysis would show that the mentally ill were experiencing longer incarcerations than others and that many of the important gains in decarceration were occurring for people who didn't need community mental health treatment.

ALL OF THESE POLICY FAILURES were reflected in the simple reality that Rikers was not an adequate treatment setting for someone as ill as Mr. Ballard. At multiple turns, his clinical signs and symptoms were met with punishment or neglect. The sicker he got, the worse he was treated. When Jake Pearson of the Associated Press reported on Mr. Ballard's death, a firestorm ensued that has continued to spread. Community mental health experts and advocates and local politicians were just soaking up the horrible details of Mr. Ballard's death when Pearson reported on another disaster, the death of Jerome Murdough in a mental observation unit in the same jail. Mr. Murdough, also seriously mentally ill, essentially baked to death when his cell overheated. We investigated these deaths and shared our findings with our boss, Health Commissioner Bassett, who found us the funding we needed to design a new type of unit—one that would mirror community settings and provide the types of care that hadn't been possible. This came just after we had gotten DOC and city officials to agree to build a clinical alternative to solitary confinement. As one would expect, the treatment innovations that were appropriate after someone with mental illness broke a jail rule were just as important before they ran afoul of those rules (and to prevent that from happening). The new mental health units were called Program for Accelerated Clinical Effectiveness (PACE). The PACE units were designed by Dr. Ford and her team, who identified several especially vulnerable cohorts of patients, the first being patients who had just returned from the hospital. The health and security staff on these units would be selected from staff who wanted to become part of a new approach, would train as a team, and would provide a full schedule of individual and group programs, including art therapy, group counseling, and traditional mental health and medical care. These units would roll out slowly, about one a year, but we quickly saw that the patients on these units had better medication adherence rates and lower rates of use of force, reflecting both the clinical improvement of the patients and the better engagement by security and health staff working as teams. As we continued to convert existing mental observation units to the PACE model, these results remained consistent, and in 2016 we received funding to expand this approach to 12 of the 30 units.

The success of the PACE units brings into high relief the failures of jails in caring for patients with serious mental illness. This success comes at a high price, however. Each PACE unit costs about $2 million more each year than a regular mental observation unit. This cost is for about 20 beds, meaning that each bed represents an additional cost of $100,000 to meet the clinical needs of these seriously mentally ill patients in jail. These costs are on top of the $168,000 annual costs per bed for DOC, yielding a cost of $268,000 for the care of patients like Mr. Ballard.[7]

If these costs seem high, they are. Community models of treatment that can mix supportive housing with both mental health and substance use treatment are not only far cheaper than jail; they're associated with fewer incarcerations.[8] In NYC, developing a model that meets these diverse needs has shown a considerable reduction in public costs, not just jail expenses.[9] But the most important statistic for city officials may be the costs of litigation. When patients like Mr. Ballard experience the health risks of incarceration in the form of injury, death, or disfigurement, there is most often a lawsuit on their behalf. NYC settled Mr. Ballard's suit for $5.75 million, enough to fund 50 supportive housing units with mental health and substance use services for a year.[10]

The horrible death of Bradley Ballard on Rikers Island signals the most extreme and tragic health risk of jail. His death also shows that the health risks of incarceration are not spread evenly among those who come to jail. The inability of the jail system to respond humanely and effectively to Mr. Ballard's mental health problems resulted in him dying a preventable medical death. Both infection and diabetes are treatable conditions. Even more minor conditions than these can result in death when the patient is isolated and neglected by health and security staff. The development of the PACE units was a critical response; they represent a new standard of care in jail mental health and fulfill an obligation to our most vulnerable patients. But most jail systems will never cobble together the resources for such high-level care, and even when these resources do materialize, keeping units such as these focused on care (instead of punishment) is extremely tough over the long term. The inexorable pressure of dual loyalty on health staff and the shifting priorities of security staff almost guarantee that seriously mentally ill patients will receive substandard care behind bars. For those who can be accommodated in community treatment, clinical outcomes and costs should guide us toward alternatives to incarceration, such as assisted outpatient treatment.

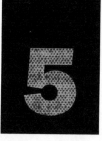

Human Rights and Correctional Health

CANDIE HAILEY CAME INTO JAIL with about the worst label possible: baby killer. In 2012, Ms. Hailey ran into a group of women she knew on the streets of the South Bronx. They exchanged words, and a fight ensued, during which the toddler of one of the women was injured, suffering a cut and a fractured skull. The women alleged that Ms. Hailey attacked them and the toddler with a knife, leading to a charge of attempted murder for Ms. Hailey, who was held in jail on $500,000 bail.[1] As she related to Jake Pearson of the Associated Press, almost every day she spent in the Rose M. Singer Center jail on Rikers would bring conflict and violence relating to this charge. A fighter by nature, Ms. Hailey did not respond to the abuses of jail meekly. During her three years in jail, Ms. Hailey would spend over two years in solitary confinement, including 27 of her first 29 months. She received her first infraction and first stay in solitary confinement in her second month of jail, for arguing over who should clean a shower. A couple of weeks later, Ms. Hailey cursed at a guard, and during the resulting physical altercation, she spit on the officer. That interaction landed her in solitary for 95 days, but the sentence was almost irrelevant. Ms. Hailey's response to the stress and violence of solitary was to act out against her surroundings, resulting in even more infractions and "box" time with each passing month. New infractions occurred for cursing officers, blocking her cell window, failing to obey commands, and splashing staff with toilet water. In some instances, Ms. Hailey would smear her cell with feces, with the mind-set that "If you're gonna treat me like a dog, I'm gonna act like one."[2]

While the experiences of Candie Hailey seem extreme, they're a foreseeable result of how correctional settings work. As paramilitary operations, jails and prisons are designed to thwart transparency and undercut any priorities that come into conflict with "security." One stark and deadly consequence of this approach is the erosion of the health mission by the security service. Almost nobody who works in corrections or correctional health ever uses the terms "dual loyalty" or "human rights," but these concepts are absolutely required to understand how preventable death and disability are so common among our patients. The essence of dual loyalty is that despite being a doctor or nurse or social worker, our individual interactions with our patients in jail or prison are influenced by the security setting around us. Most of the time, dual loyalty exerts a mild influence that we might not notice, such as rethinking writing an order for an asthma inhaler (which requires front- instead of rear-cuffing) or for a cane (which could be used as a weapon). Maybe the most dramatic and tortured aspect of dual loyalty in correctional health is clearance for solitary confinement. This process, which occurs at almost every American jail and prison, is at the core of human rights problems in correctional health, and the influence is not just on individual providers but also on the overall functioning of every correctional health service.

One of the striking features of Ms. Hailey's case is how the health service responded to obvious and repeated health emergencies and crises. During the 27 months of constant solitary, Ms. Hailey also at times inflicted violence against herself. She repeatedly swallowed odd objects, cut herself, and hit her head on the walls. These acts of self-harm elicited medical treatments for the injuries, mental health evaluations, and brief periods on suicide watch. In virtually every encounter with health staff, her actions were judged to be manipulative, aimed at escaping solitary confinement. These assessments give us a glimpse of the core of dual loyalty and how it erodes the health mission in jails and prisons. Health staff are asked to decide whether acts of self-harm are true suicide attempts or not. If their clinical assessment is that the patient was not suicidal or psychotic, then the patient is essentially found fit to be in solitary. For patients with schizophrenia or bipolar disease, the response was more clear-cut: these patients could be removed from solitary and then treated in the hospital. But few hospitals would admit patients like Ms. Hailey, at least for more than a day or two. This left the jail to manage her behaviors and the mental health staff to choose between the only options presented: was she a malingerer or a psychotic patient who needed urgent mental health care? It's an absurd binary and does nobody any good.

DUAL LOYALTY IN CORRECTIONAL HEALTH has been written about in the past by people outside jails and prisons, including my own current organization, Physicians for Human Rights.[3] These reports have identified the caustic impact that security priorities can have on health staff, but these discussions have been largely absent from the operations of correctional health, where the problem exists essentially unchecked. Inside the walls of US jails and prisons, dual loyalty is so widespread and accepted that only when a patient dies are questions asked. Generally, there is a quick response to condemn an individual nurse or doctor for failing to do their job, but with no discussion of the pressures that led them and thousands of others to stray from the path of patient care. Some of the most shocking cases involve patients who die while being restrained in a chair or being held in a cell, but who are under medical "monitoring." These cases often reveal that health staff cease acting in the best interests of the patient because their frame of reference is driven by the security perspective. The 2013 death of Christopher Lopez in Colorado's San Carolos Prison is one of these instances. Mr. Lopez, a schizophrenic, was sentenced to two years in prison for trespassing but had an additional four years (with extensive solitary confinement) added to his sentence for assaulting a corrections officer while in prison. During his stints in and out of solitary, Mr. Lopez acquired the label of being a noncompliant patient and one who required "special controls," meaning enhanced restraints. On the day of his death, Mr. Lopez refused to obey a command to move toward the door of his cell. This seemingly minor act of defiance (or misunderstanding) can be perceived as a serious sign of disrespect by security staff. As a result of Mr. Lopez's inaction, a probe team entered the cell with riot gear, restrained him, and placed him in a special restraint chair with a spit mask over his face. Medical staff were present for this episode and participated by administering psychotropic medication and remaining in the cell with security staff. Video of this episode shows Mr. Lopez having a grand mal seizure while health and security staff watch and do nothing more than place him on the ground when he becomes unresponsive. At some point during the video, health staff can be heard asking Mr. Lopez, "What are you doing? Why are you doing this? I can see you breathing." After another 30 minutes of unresponsiveness, health staff discovered that Mr. Lopez had stopped breathing, and they initiated CPR.[4] These cases of jail patients dying in full view of health staff are tragically common. Shortly after leaving Rikers, I reviewed the case of a young man who died in similar tragic circumstances in the St. Luis Obispo jail. This 36-year-old man, Andrew Holland, a longtime mental health patient, also met his death after 48 hours in a restraint chair while health staff administered meaningless interventions.[5]

Even when health staff are not actively part of causing a death, they may shy away from doing their jobs in critical situations. One such case involved the 2010 death of a schizophrenic inmate, Leonard Strickland, in New York's Clinton State Prison. Nothing was known publicly about the case until the *New York Times* reported on the death and obtained video showing correction officers dragging a lifeless Mr. Strickland across the floor after a brutal use of force within clear view of a nurse. As Mr. Strickland lay on the floor close to death, with the nurse standing to the side, Department of Correction officers continued to yell "Stop resisting!"[6] In 2014 I saw a patient newly arrived from the same prison system with a similar story. He reported being assaulted over several days by a group of corrections officers, and when he arrived at Rikers, he essentially fell out of the bus with serious injuries and was transported directly to the hospital. He related to me that during the several days of assaults he was taken to a jail clinic, where the health staff never asked him how he became injured, but instead asked the corrections officers how they should document the cause of injuries in the medical records.

In 2012, we published a paper in which we asserted that without integrating core human rights and medical ethics concepts like dual loyalty into the correctional health mission, the health service would fail.[7] Our position then (and now) was that even with great correctional health staff, the right policies and procedures, and plenty of resources, the nature of corrections is to wear away medical decision making and to bend the health service into a tool of the security service. Over a year, we developed a structure for incorporating human rights into our health system, including practical tools like assessments of deficiencies linked to human rights issues and a human rights quality improvement committee. Our first project, a dual loyalty assessment based on staff and patient interviews, as well as reviews of patient records, led us to develop a dual loyalty training for all health staff. Ms. Hailey came into the jail system as we were embarking on this work, and her experiences reveal the failures of the health service to act on her behalf.

In health care, we understand that patients with behavioral health problems like borderline or narcissistic personality disorder may not be truthful and may act inappropriately. As a medical student, I can recall the oversimplified description of personality disorders being clustered into categories of patients who were excessively "wild, weird, and worried." Later, as a resident at Montefiore, I can recall seeing a clinic walk-in patient for a simple complaint about his eyes, at which point he launched into a fantastic and angry story about how his eyes moved around in his head every night and our clinic had ignored his complaints. I asked a series of questions about the concerns he had with his eyes, as well as a standard set of questions about his overall health. Unlike other patients I'd cared for who were psychotic or having some other profound decompensation, this patient seemed to understand and appreciate the world around him, but in that first encounter I felt overwhelmed by the story he was telling me and his aggressive and threatening demeanor. When I presented this patient to my preceptor, Dr. Joe Deluca, he quickly focused on how the patient and I had interacted, starting with, "How did you feel sitting in the room with him?" I told him that after a few minutes I felt like my skin was on fire and I wanted to bolt out of the exam room. "That's what happens when a patient with a personality disorder runs into a doctor who doesn't see it," he replied. His counsel was for me to take this patient on as my own and see him more often than I normally would. After a couple of months following this plan, the patient and I settled into a rhythm of shared expectations about what we would cover in each session, and his concerns about his eyes gave way to some other health issues that he hadn't ever sought care for. Importantly, the way I felt on my initial encounter with him could have cemented the dynamic between us, which would have led me to dread every further contact with him as a patient. Also, not knowing how to process the strongly negative emotional response I had to him during that first encounter would have led me to focus on the eye complaint being false and to ratchet up my assessment about him being a malingerer or a liar.

This dynamic is central to the mission of mental health professionals, but for those of us in primary care and medical specialties, it's easy to ignore or sidestep our own emotional responses to patients when they aren't truthful, and these dynamics are critical to whether the patient gets good or bad care from us. Those of us fortunate enough to train with mentors like Dr. Deluca learn that fantastic stories and aggressive demeanor are often part of a patient's accumulated trauma and mental health status. We fail as doctors when we take these interactions personally and don't integrate them into our clinical formulation. But in jail, this approach to understanding the patient is often undercut by pervasive focus on punishment. Health staff find themselves advocating for punishment, sometimes as a prerequisite to clinical treatment, even when that punishment is solitary confinement. This is essentially where Ms. Hailey found herself in the jails. As she had difficult encounters with health and security staff alike, she was locked into adversarial dynamics that hardened over time.

I was once chatting with a patient who had considerable mental health issues, on the same solitary confinement unit that Ms. Hailey was on. An experienced mental health staffer approached us and said to her, "Tell him what you did to be in there, and why you have to stay in there a little longer before you can come out to group [therapy]." This punishment mentality is unfortunately pervasive among correctional health staff and their leadership. In 2011, my boss, Dr. Amanda Parsons, and I were listening to a pitch from a for-profit correctional health group interested in providing care in the NYC jails. Their medical director told us about a great new diabetes quality improvement project that he'd implemented in a local jail. Basically, patients were informed of their plan of care, and part of their incentive to participate was that they would be referred to security staff for infractions if they didn't participate. On a different occasion, I visited another jurisdiction's mental health lockup with Health Commissioner Mary Bassett and our medical director, Dr. Ross MacDonald. We observed in horror as mental health staff used their "treatment team" meeting to refer patients for infractions with security staff. This co-opting of health staff for the security mission erodes the ability of the health staff to really see their patients objectively and is unfortunately more the norm than the exception in US correctional health settings.

Dual loyalty also flourishes because even small measures of independence of health staff can be eroded and dominated by the security perspective. One Sunday afternoon I received a call that a patient had died in our medical infirmary. This wasn't an altogether unheard-of event, since we housed some of our sickest patients in the infirmary. But the call I received indicated that the patient, Ronald Spear, who was sick enough to require hemodialysis to live, had been involved in a use of force. I headed into Rikers and, once there, found the deceased on the floor, DOC setting up an investigation, and a very different set of stories on what had happened. I focused on the care he'd received before his death, while the DOC investigators and Bronx NYPD homicide detective on the scene took over the official investigation into the use of force. The story that would emerge was that Mr. Spear had a verbal altercation with a DOC officer that escalated to pushing. The DOC officer then punched him in the face and slammed him to the ground, kicking him in the head several times before kneeling over his body and snarling, "Remember that I'm the one who did this to you."[8] This happened in our infirmary, not in some faraway intake pen, reminding everyone involved that there was no part of the jails that wasn't controlled by security staff. For health staff weighing how much to advocate for a patient, these types of reminders often serve to tip the balance away from standing up for a patient and toward the corrosive effect of dual loyalty.

Ms. Hailey's actions during her time in the solitary unit can be viewed as part of her mental health issues, but they can also be viewed as basic survival instincts. The stress of solitary confinement can drive anyone to extreme behaviors in an attempt to escape their cell, even for a short ride to the hospital or transfer to the jail clinic. These actions often escalate as the patients are labeled as malingering or goal oriented and need to take more and more extreme actions to achieve the same result. Both security and health staff become numbed to the physical and mental toll that this setting takes on patients. Five Omar Mualimm-ak, a friend and colleague, once spent over five years in the box both in Rikers and upstate in the New York prison system for nonviolent infractions. He writes,

> There was no touch. My food was pushed through a slot. Doors were activated by buzzers, even the one that led to a literal cage directly outside of my cell for one hour per day of "recreation." Even time had no meaning in the SHU. The lights were kept on for 24 hours. I often found myself

wondering if an event I was recollecting had happened that morning or days before. I talked to myself. I began to get scared that the guards would come in and kill me and leave me hanging in the cell. Who would know if something happened to me? Just as I was invisible, so was the space I inhabited. The very essence of life, I came to learn during those seemingly endless days, is human contact, and the affirmation of existence that comes with it. Losing that contact, you lose your sense of identity. You become nothing.[9]

Mr. Mualimm-ak now runs a nonprofit organization focused on advocating for the millions of people currently and formerly incarcerated in the United States. For him, even healthcare encounters were so depersonalized that they didn't bring relief from the isolation of solitary confinement. "For the five years I spent in the box, I received insulin shots for my diabetes by extending my arm through the food slot in the cell's door. ('Therapy' for prisoners with mental illness is often conducted this way, as well.) One day, the person who gave me the shot yanked roughly on my arm through the small opening and I instinctively pulled back. This earned me another ticket for 'refusing medical attention,' adding additional time to my solitary sentence." Mr. Mualimm-ak became one of the core advisors to our human rights agenda in the correctional health service, and he repeatedly identified the tangled roles our health staff played in solitary confinement units like the one Ms. Hailey was held in as the epicenter of human rights and dual loyalty concerns.

Beyond the psychological stress of solitary confinement, these settings often had deplorable physical conditions. In Ms. Hailey's unit flies often swarmed in the solitary cells, with patients constantly swatting them away. Sometimes a patient would block their toilet, either in protest of something specific or through general frustration, and water and sewage would flow into neighboring cells. Patients on these units would smear their own feces inside the cells in acts of protest. Plumbing repairs were often slow in coming, and they were quickly undone. In my work I have encountered a fair number of patients who smeared—every one of them in a solitary cell. This act alone should help us consider just how extreme the human response to solitary confinement can be. The deplorable conditions and human suffering create indelible memories for anyone with experience on these units.

The loss of trust between correctional patients and health providers is the central consequence of dual loyalty, and it leads to considerable avoidable morbidity and mortality. The labeling that Ms. Hailey experienced virtually guaranteed that health staff would lack objectivity in their assessments and care. One of the enduring truths of our case reviews is that once a patient receives a label as a malingerer or otherwise problematic patient, it's extremely unlikely that staff will approach him or her objectively. One of the most profound dual loyalty cases I ever saw was that of a man injured during a use of force. His hip was fractured, and the patient was seen by a nurse and told that he would need to go directly to the hospital. The doctor who saw him was told by security staff that he was faking his symptoms and that he just wanted to go to the hospital. In the part of the doctor's note that recorded the physical examination, there was a textbook description of a fracture: limb shortening and rotation. But in the assessment/plan part of the note, the doctor wrote that there was unclear evidence of hip fracture and that the patient should be put into a wheelchair and taken in a van to the X-ray on Rikers. This plan was impossible because of the pain involved in sitting in a wheelchair, and it was also completely unnecessary given the information gathered by the doctor. The provider's mind was made up by information from the security service rather than the patient's actual signs and symptoms.

During Ms. Hailey's incarceration, we opened the Clinical Alternative to Punitive Segregation unit for seriously mentally ill patients. We had succeeded in eliminating solitary for one vulnerable group. But because Ms. Hailey wasn't assessed as being seriously mentally ill, she spent limited time in this new unit. My own knowledge of her case came when two dedicated patient advocates took up her cause. Jennifer Parrish, director of the Urban Justice Center's Mental Health project, and Jane Stanicki of Hour Children both began to visit with her regularly and provided feedback about the care she and others required and the conditions on the women's solitary unit. Our own director of projects, Cecilia Flaherty, joined in the regular visits to this unit, working with the mental health staff of Corizon and the security staff to try to maximize out-of-cell time and access to group therapy and other programs. These visits brought some improved conditions and a touch of humanity to the women viewed as most problematic, but they also revealed how toxic the solitary unit was to our own staff and their relationships with their patients. We had asked staff to work in these units for years without preparing them for the realities of dual loyalty or providing the tools to address these concerns. Without support or training, health staff followed the lead of their security colleagues for guidance on how to interact with patients. In retrospect, this shouldn't have been a surprise. Security staff were the ones who protected health staff and allowed them to provide care. Health staff would stop me or Cecilia with the same complaints as the security staff had: "You're being manipulated by these women," or "They're lying to you and just trying to get out of their punishment." While it was true that many of these and other patients didn't tell the truth or worked to split the staff against each other, being in the jail setting brought out the same type of moral judgment from health staff that we often saw in the DOC staff.

Ultimately, Ms. Hailey was found innocent of the charges against her, and she returned to the community, having accumulated an unimaginable amount of trauma and depersonalization during her three years of incarceration. She struggled to reacclimate to life outside the jail. Ms. Hailey has attended several oversight meetings held by the New York City Board of Correction and spoken on the horrible experiences and consequences of solitary confinement. At one of her appearances, Ms. Hailey reported that she tried to kill herself on a regular basis, but that staff ignored her and treated her like an animal.[10]

Incorporating human rights into the health operation of the jails has taken us down an uneven but rewarding path. As we learned more about injuries and solitary confinement, it became clear that we needed to develop a structured response to the observation that the jail setting sometimes harms our patients. While our mission was to assess and reduce the health risks of incarceration, this was not a mission welcomed by those around us in the security service, city government, or even all of the health service. Many of our senior team had learned to conduct forensic evaluations of torture survivors at Montefiore, so that asylum seekers could bring medical evidence of abuse into their asylum hearing. This type of human rights training was critical to our view of the problems, but documenting abuse that occurred thousands of miles away and years earlier is a far cry from seeing and documenting problems down the hall, with patients who are confined to their sites of abuse. As the leaders of the jail health service, we were on the inside of this system, and we immediately sensed the many layers of cultural and political resistance to our focus on human rights as a part of the health mission.

One challenge to the human rights construct was that it didn't always track with how American health systems address problems. Healthcare improvement in the United States is built on a standardized approach that relies on finding and fixing problems. For individual patients, there's something called a SOAP note that is used across health care, with "SOAP" standing for "Subjective, Objective, Assessment, and Plan." The notion is that we ask for the patient's input in the subjective part of the encounter, then get our own objective data from sources such as a physical exam and vital signs, followed by our assessment (usually the diagnoses), and then formulate a plan. At the macro level, health systems are set up to find and address health problems quickly, because any delay in acting can cause morbidity or mortality. All of this makes sense. Even how we improve things in health care is action oriented. We use quality assurance processes to look for problems in almost every area of care and quality improvement interventions to come up with new workflows, policies, and trainings to fix those problems.

Juxtapose these systems to human rights, where the initial step of identifying and documenting a problem is sometimes the only measure that can be taken for a while. In my new position at Physician for Human Rights, I've spent a fair amount of time in Iraq and Bangladesh working on the abuses suffered by the Yazidi and Rohingya, respectively. In that work, we're focused on documenting the truth of mass crimes committed against these ethnic minorities, and our hopes for accountability are pretty far down the road. In Syria we document attack after attack on hospitals and doctors, and it's unclear when there will be any accountability for those war crimes. But without accountability there can't be any justice, so we and others work to collect forensic evidence, and in places like Rwanda and Yugoslavia, there has been some recent accountability. The killing fields of Northern Iraq and Rakhine Myanmar are certainly worlds away from Rikers Island, but every correctional health system needs the capacity to document abuses that they may not be able to address. Unfortunately, without correctional health leaders who believe in the human rights imperative, this critical work is sadly but quickly scrubbed out from these systems.

The challenge of providers buying into human rights isn't just about the speed with which the problems can be fixed, however. Health care is an industry and culture that has its own language, and introducing a new set of principles requires using accepted language. As we developed a structure in 2011 to focus our work on human rights, our first practical move was to create a human rights quality improvement committee. This simple action mated the new ideas of human rights to the quality improvement apparatus that was already viewed as credible by our health staff. This group is composed of senior clinical and operational staff, and the first issue the committee identified was the need for an assessment of dual loyalty in our health service. Before that, there was an echoing silence around dual loyalty in correctional health. We knew that it was omnipresent, but there was no evidence, because it had never been addressed. The assessment would focus on where it was most pervasive. To assess dual loyalty, we looked at the interaction between health staff and their patients who were held in solitary confinement. First, we analyzed the medical notes of 24 patients in solitary.[11] All told, those patients had 5,602 medical notes. Among them, we found 651 (12.2%) notes that included work or comments that were not in the patient's interest—the definition of health care's vulnerability to dual loyalty. The most common finding (312 notes) was that the patient's behaviors were "goal directed" or exhibiting "secondary gain" to influence their housing status. One note read, "Inmate is well known to mental health and all recent notes indicate he is threatening to harm himself if put in a cell. He owes 109 punitive segregation days and wants to be placed in [clinic]. He has reported that he will swallow a razor, batteries, cut himself, etc., if placed in a cell. He is at high risk for repeating self-injurious gestures to get himself moved, but low risk for actual suicide." These results laid out the false dichotomy that our staff were trapped in, trying to use their clinical skills to decipher whether someone was harming themselves just because they wanted out of solitary or because they were really mentally ill. Putting aside the fact that being a mental health provider isn't the same as being a lie detector, we found that staff perceived the "goal-oriented" actions of people who just wanted out of solitary as not worrisome and the actions of psychotic or otherwise more mentally ill people as more serious. The death of Jason Echevarria helped to put the lie to this distinction. He was certainly engaged in a goal-oriented act, and he died nonetheless.

Our next step to characterize our dual loyalty concerns was to host a series of focus groups with mental health staff. These sessions revealed that over one-third of these providers felt that their work regularly caused them to compromise their ethics (higher than the 24% of other health staff) and that their work in solitary was not real mental health work and damaged their relationships with patients. These staff reported that working in a setting where they were part of punishing a patient, or where they sometimes couldn't deliver evidence-based care, damaged their identity as healthcare providers. Mental health staff who clear patients for solitary confinement feel the weight of participating in this process. One mental health staff member reported, "Even though I am not a believer in solitary confinement as punishment, I sometimes feel that the least harmful path is to return a personality disordered person to solitary in this scenario. This is very personally distressing to me and situations like this leave me with a negative impression of the work I do and my workplace."[12]

Our final step in the dual loyalty assessment was to have qualitative interviews with 19 patients who had committed self-harm, mainly in attempts to get out of solitary or to protest against conditions in solitary. These patients viewed the health service as deeply compromised in its ability to provide actual medical care to them. One patient reported, "The doctor is not for us, [security staff] influence them [mental health staff] to clear people who are not supposed to be cleared." Another patient reported that he was "afraid of being in a cell alone and says his fear of being alone in his cell . . . will lead him to try to cut and hang himself as well as ingest soap whenever possible."[13]

With this information in hand, we set about developing a training for all clinical staff on the issues of dual loyalty. We created an online module that introduced dual loyalty and other human rights concepts through a series of clinical scenarios that had actually occurred in our jail. Staff were given options for how to address the scenarios and were asked for feedback based on their own experiences. The scenarios included a patient whom DOC wanted to punish with solitary confinement despite having harmed himself in the past when punished this way, a request from a patient for condoms in jail (which is allowable by policy), and an incident in which a patient reports different causes of an injury than correctional officers. In the injury report scenario, a patient was in a clinic cubicle, with correctional staff insisting that he sign a form that stated he had been injured in a fight with another inmate, while he complained to the doctor that he had been injured by a guard. In this circumstance, the doctor was able to note the patient's version in our electronic medical record without the correction officer knowing so that it was referred to us at the senior level, defusing the immediate pressure. A total of 93 percent of respondents indicated that they had encountered or heard of this type of scenario. The final scenario involved patients being brought into the jail clinic restrained on stretchers and being beaten by correction officers in full view of health staff (see chap. 2). When asked for possible responses to this scenario, one health staffer reported, "Tell DOC staff this is highly inappropriate and threaten to report this to all higher authorities in which their jobs may be in jeopardy. Such beatings (if done at all) should never take place in public." A total of 16 percent of respondents indicated that they had encountered or heard of a similar event.

This scenario raised the persistent issue of our stretchers being used to restrain inmates for abuse. Every jail clinic has a stretcher with emergency gear, such as defibrillators and oxygen tanks, so that we can respond to emergencies outside the clinic. Like one would see in hospitals, nursing staff check the equipment every day and note that everything is present and functional. In the jails, DOC staff occasionally come into the clinic and grab our stretcher to take out for their own use, usually to restrain an unruly inmate. In these circumstances, they don't call a medical emergency or ask for our staff to accompany them. Not only do we lose our stretcher so that we can't respond to emergencies, but our medical equipment is also used for unclear purposes, sometimes including outright assault of restrained patients.[14] As long as I've worked in the jail system, we've worked to get DOC to stop this practice, and despite unending memos and reminders from their senior leadership, the practice continues. When this happens, our stretcher usually turns up in a random part of the jail hours or days later, sometimes damaged, making it impossible for us to properly respond to true medical emergencies in the interim. Early in my tenure, I got one of these calls from a jail about a stretcher being taken by DOC staff. I went to the jail and found a probe team of about 10 officers in riot gear headed down the hallway with our stretcher. I stood in the middle of the hallway and signaled to the captain that they needed to return the stretcher. After he and I barked back and forth and his officers threw a few remarks my way, he relented and gave it back, and I wheeled the stretcher away under the glare of the probe team.

After taking the stretcher to the clinic, I went to the housing area where the officers were headed and found a restrained patient on the ground, kicking and with officers standing around. It was clear that the officers needed a safe way to transport this person, and I made the humbling decision to go get the stretcher myself and bring it back for the officers to use to transport the patient to the jail intake. I ran and got the stretcher and suffered a long 15 minutes of insults from the officers for sticking my nose into their business. Afterward, I directed our staff to give our old stretchers to DOC so they could have their own transport option that didn't harm our ability to respond to medical emergencies. The risk that these stretchers would be used for nefarious purposes didn't escape me, but the reality was that DOC did seem to have a legitimate need to transport people who had been restrained. But today many of these stretchers remain unused, and the security staff continue to take our stretchers when they want them.

Near the end of my time at Rikers, I encountered a glimmer of hope on this front, though: I responded to an emergency in a hallway where an agitated patient, who had just been teargassed, was on the floor, rear-cuffed and yelling that he couldn't breathe. He was surrounded by a probe team of security staff, and when I approached with our stretcher, DOC simultaneously rolled in with one of the stretchers that we had given them. Because the patient was stating that he couldn't breathe, I asked DOC to back off so I could get him up and on our stretcher to go directly to the clinic. Unfortunately, a week later, I received word that DOC staff had returned to their practice of grabbing our stretcher for nonmedical use instead of using the one we'd given them. The stretcher issue is a good indicator of how imbalanced the power dynamic is, and how sticking up for our independence as a health service can bring us into conflict with security staff and their own needs. DOC managers should train and equip their staff to transport unruly people without removing essential medical equipment, but the low priority of the health mission and lack of effective management of DOC allow this problem to persist.

Our dual loyalty trainings revealed another disconnect closer to home: the cultural differences between human rights and medicine. The first lesson of human rights is to document everything, even when there's no prospect for change or accountability. This is a tough sell for doctors and nurses who want to diagnose, treat, and resolve every issue they encounter.

This disconnect is amplified when documenting or reporting abuse comes at a personal price. One staffer reported, "Part of dual loyalty is threats from DOC if we go above and beyond to protect a patient. We are then in a position that the officer may take 'extra long' to respond to medical staff being assaulted by a patient due to medical staff reporting human rights violations. We have to bear in mind the safety of the patient as well as our own safety."

A central effort in our attempt to solve the problems of dual loyalty has been to improve our EMR to allow us to better monitor vulnerable groups of patients and their health outcomes.[15] As a primary care doctor, I was ambivalent about the arrival of EMRs in clinic settings because their benefits came with some important downsides. For anyone who has sat with a doctor who was focused on a screen instead of them, these drawbacks are well known. This is even more of an issue in jails, where getting health providers to pay attention to the human being in front of them is a major challenge. But as a human rights tool, I have never encountered anything so powerful. Having an EMR that we could change ourselves allowed us to match variables associated with vulnerable cohorts of patients with other risk factors of the jail setting and with health outcomes we cared about. We took this approach in tracking injuries, including blows to the head. We also took this approach with self-harm. We were able to create standard templates in the EMR that would capture structured data elements about each patient who experienced these important health outcomes, including types of injuries and self-harm acts, as well as clinical severity. We could also capture key information about the jail setting. For self-harm, we could capture type of housing area (solitary confinement, mental health, general population), time of day, and location in the jails. For injuries, we could capture whether the injury was intentional, and if so, who caused the injury—a correction officer or someone else. By capturing the characteristics of the patients, their health outcomes, and the jail setting together, we could then make powerful analyses of these data in the aggregate. In these ways, the EMR has allowed us to change how we collect data to improve individual clinical encounters, but it has also allowed for analysis of the risks of incarceration. We've generated numerous reports on these topics, often with the idea that they would be reviewed and acted upon even by people outside the health service. This represents the crux of our human rights work. Some of the risks of incarceration we could address ourselves, by improving our provision of care. Others would require outside intervention, including investigation of abuse and neglect and rethinking decisions about who should be incarcerated in the first place.

Candie Hailey's case and our data reveal the troubling experience of health staff clearing patients for solitary confinement. When jails and prisons seek to place someone in solitary confinement, mental health staff are often asked to certify that they won't suffer some serious harm as a result of being punished in this manner. This task is different than being able to pull people out who become ill. It essentially asks a health professional to guarantee that an individual can be subjected to punishment in solitary without suffering harm. Health clearance for solitary is not based on any reliable science and violates basic medical ethics principles, because, of course, that patient is supposed to suffer. It's punishment, after all.[16] Also, it is unfortunately one of the few correctional practices that continues to be supported by both security officials and some advocates for prisoner's rights. Security leaders (and city or county law departments) want a medical seal of approval for their punishments, to absolve them from liability for later adverse outcomes. Some lawyers and other advocates for prisoner's rights also press for this clearance to be part of oversight of solitary, incorrectly thinking that this helps patients. It does not. Because there is no medical science behind this work, health staff cannot predict the future any better than anyone else. Health staff in this role find themselves in the path of the security staff just at the moment when they want to punish. The outcome of this dynamic is predetermined: the more powerful security staff will prevail in most cases, and the health staff will learn to stay out of the way. Advocates and judges who promote this practice then become frustrated with health staff for not using their power to keep patients out of solitary when appropriate, not understanding that consigning health providers into an unscientific and unethical process helps to create this fictional capacity. In general, when we raise this issue with security leaders, oversight bodies, and advocates, it is seen as ethical hand-wringing. The fear of liability for sending the wrong patients into solitary is the primary concern. The nature of the clearance process undermines medical ethics and guts our ability to provide care. And the other side of the balance sheet is blank; the thing everyone wants, a safe approach to solitary confinement, remains mythological. It is one fiction in support of another.

We've failed to win the argument and get out of the dirty business of solitary clearance, so we seek to reduce the harm of the process, especially on the line staff and in their interactions with patients. In addition to barring solitary punishment of adolescents and the mentally ill, DOC in NYC also undertook significant reforms to reduce the use of solitary among adults. All of this shrunk the footprint of our clearance and dual loyalty issues. More recently, we have started to shift responsibility from the line staff to leadership for the clearance process, with the goal of keeping the facility staff out of the ethical compromise and keeping them engaged with their patients in a manner that's true to their training and mission. This also removes the facility staff from being stuck in the heat of the moment, when security staff urgently want a clearance sheet signed and ask health staff to divine the potential health outcomes of solitary. In our higher-level reviews, we rely on data (see chap. 3), and instead of saying that someone is cleared, we record that there is a health risk for everyone who enters solitary and that the patient in question has either the baseline health risk when exposed to solitary or a higher-than-baseline risk. It's important to remember that clearance is different from surveillance, which is an actual health process. All solitary confinement settings that exist should have health staff present every day to detect patients who are faring poorly for medical or mental health reasons. These patients should be removed, and they should receive all the assessments and care they need. This is a true health intervention, and it does not make the health service part of the decision to punish. The pressures of the security service still bear on the health staff, and patients will surely be motivated to get out of any facilities that cause them harm. In the end, there is no way to balance human rights and solitary confinement. We need to eliminate reliance on solitary as a method of punishment. For correctional health staff, being the stamp of approval for punishment is far more caustic and unscientific than being asked to identify and care for those who need removal from solitary.

ESTABLISHING HUMAN RIGHTS as part of our health mission has revealed how complex a setting we work in. There is no doubt that the issues of dual loyalty, confidentiality, abuse, and neglect are fundamental challenges to the health of incarcerated people. Every correctional health service needs the support and autonomy to deliver care to patients and also to train staff regarding these issues. Ideally, the correctional health service can discuss and address these issues with the security authority, such as the sheriff or DOC. Many will correctly point out that the health service is always less powerful than (and often employed by) the security service, making a meaningful collaborative approach difficult to achieve. Because the dual loyalty trainings capture feedback, we have learned a great deal from our staff about how to navigate these power imbalances. In the scenario where the patient disputed the cause of his injury, the doctor was able to document the truth of the patient's injury in the EMR but still avoid a conflict with the correction officers in the moment. This can be tricky when a doctor is seeing a patient in a small cubicle and with an officer standing near or at the entrance to the cubicle. Although it's bad practice, the officer standing at the ready may be the same person who just fought with the patient, and their animosity can simmer and come to a second boil while the doctor or nurse is trying to deliver care. I have been in the middle of a number of fights between officers and patients, and worry about being harmed is a common concern. Also, the health providers have often been told something about the patient by DOC staff before the patient is ever seen, so there's often an expectation that the doctor or nurse will treat the patient in a manner in which the officer dictates. I've had officers tell me that a patient was faking, or that he or she threw the first punch, or had it coming, along with a number of other comments designed to color the interaction with the patient.

As a result, building out the capacity of our EMR to receive and report sensitive information relating to abuse helped to keep health staff out of adversarial interactions with security staff. The more we can build systems to alert us of key events like broken bones or lacerations and aggregate data for larger systems-level discussions, the more transparent the system is and the less room there is for ignoring problems. Also, reporting on standard metrics like injury and self-harm rates, as well as how reliably our patients are brought to their appointments, can give both oversight bodies and security and health leaders a common set of metrics to track.

These issues are rarely discussed in US correctional health systems, and the fact that human rights and dual loyalty remain basically off-limits topics in most jails and prisons reflects the deep divide between our highest principles and the base reality that Candie Hailey experienced. Staff and patients alike are thirsty for a more meaningful approach. These trainings were very popular with staff: over 600 health staff completed the online module, and more than 90 percent of them reported that the trainings were helpful and that they wanted more similar opportunities.

There is no doubt that correctional health services can either protect or erode an inmate's human rights. On most days, for most staff and patients, it isn't the most critical issue. But like handwashing and infection control, ignoring human rights virtually guarantees that correctional health systems will fail their patients. Virtually every doctor and nurse is required to take yearly infection control training to ensure that they are aware of the widespread prevalence of germs in hospitals and the continual risk of spreading disease to sick patients in their care. These trainings acknowledge the presence of germs and focus on how to reduce their spread and the likelihood that health staff will harm patients through poor infection control practices. Throughout the 5,000 US jails and prisons, dual loyalty and other human rights challenges pose a similar threat, pervasive and more deadly when ignored. Like Ms. Hailey, thousands of correctional health patients manage to get into a cubicle with a doctor, nurse, or social worker, only to find out that their story isn't believed or that the provider's mind was made up before they even sat down.

Some of the conditions that Ms. Hailey experienced have improved: I left as a progressive new warden took over in the women's jail and essentially eliminated solitary confinement for women. We made minor changes to our dual loyalty trainings to meet requirements of the new settlement agreement between NYC and the US Department of Justice around brutality in the jails. Having this training now carry the weight of a DOJ settlement has helped us to establish its credibility with those outside our worldview. Before the DOJ came to NYC, we were the only jail system training our staff on dual loyalty, and our efforts were viewed as interesting and even admirable but not necessary. I think that NYC is still alone in these trainings, but since they are supported by a settlement with the DOJ, they have a higher profile and are more likely to be adopted by other systems that find themselves in trouble and looking for measures to improve health outcomes and reduce brutality. One place outside the NYC jails where this training has taken hold is in the Icahn School of Medicine at Mount Sinai, where students receive dual loyalty training, including correctional health scenarios, under the leadership of Professor Holly Atkinson. In the NYC jails, we also opened new units for women with serious mental illness that provide higher levels of therapy and support, as well as new crisis intervention teams of health and security staff to respond to confrontations and behavioral problems with the mandate to de-escalate, not escalate. These teams are standard in community policing reforms, and this approach is extremely important to reducing the escalation of frustrations into infractions, assaults, and other bad outcomes in jails. We are just now designing new units that focus on patients with personality disorders, those with profound behavioral problems. Unlike the existing units for patients with psychotic disorders, the patients on these units won't be expected to have dramatic responses because their behavioral health problems simply don't respond very well to medicines. These units will require intense work to engage with patients during group and individual therapy, and success will be far from perfect. Many of these patients experience multiple violent interactions with guards each month. The new units will hopefully help them live with less friction with staff and other patients.

In addition to training correctional health staff about human rights, we need to do more to ensure the independence of these health staff. In most jails, correctional health staff actually work for the sheriff, DOC, or a for-profit vendor hired by the security authority. We need to promote alternative models, especially in smaller places that lack the resources of NYC, Chicago, and Dallas. This will be difficult, however, because most community health systems are terrified to become involved in correctional health, and we have yet to scale up any corrections-specific nonprofit providers. In a later chapter I will discuss the prospect of bringing in Medicaid funds to cover some of the jail health care. This funding would support evidence-based care and bring welcome quality oversight that could help the health service to act more independently.

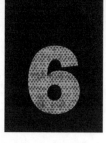

Race

Kalief Browder

KALIEF BROWDER WAS 16 when he was arrested in the Bronx. Walking home from a party along Arthur Avenue with a friend, several police cars swarmed toward them, one containing a man who reported being robbed of his backpack. Kalief and his friend said that they hadn't done anything and showed their empty pockets to prove the point. Then the story changed, and the victim in the police cruiser said that he had been robbed weeks earlier, not that night. He identified Kalief and his friend as the culprits. Both of them were arrested and arraigned on robbery and assault changes. Kalief received bail of $3,000, which his family could not raise. The high bail stemmed from a prior guilty plea in a joyriding case, for which he was given a "youthful offender" status and probation. In every state except for New York and North Carolina, this series of events likely would have resulted in either a referral back to community probation or detention in a juvenile facility. But New York and North Carolina are the two remaining states where 16- and 17-year-olds are routinely remanded to the adult jail system while they await trial. A reform movement known as "Raise the Age" hopes to end this practice but hadn't even started in earnest when Kalief was arrested.[1] Within 24 hours of being stopped on the street, Kalief Browder made the frightening journey across the bridge to Rikers Island in a Department of Correction bus. He was headed to the Robert N. Davoren Complex (RNDC), the notorious jail for adolescents, where Christopher Robinson was killed two years earlier in an attack sanctioned by correction officers.[2] The depth of brutality in this jail would prompt investigation by the US Department of Justice, which would find that "adolescent inmates at Rikers are not adequately protected from harm, including serious physical harm from the rampant use of unnecessary and excessive force by DOC staff."[3] In her description of Kalief's case in the *New Yorker*, Jennifer Gonnerman documents the violent and chaotic setting Kalief was dropped into.[4] His housing area was controlled by gangs who seemed to operate with the open acquiescence of security staff, and the only way to survive was to keep to himself and then fight when challenged. For newly arriving adolescents, there was an immediate need to establish a pecking order. That meant frequent challenges and brutal fights.

This dynamic was first revealed to me with the death of Christopher Robinson in RNDC in 2008. For him, the consequences of not fitting into this hierarchy of housing area violence were fatal. In his case, correction officers in RNDC openly conspired with a group of inmates to extort, assault, and otherwise abuse adolescents in the jail. This conspiracy was widely known as "The Program" and involved both correction officers actively participating in crimes and others turning a blind eye. Christopher Robinson resisted the efforts by this group to extort money from him, and consequently he was beaten to death in his cell. Two correction officers who participated in the homicide were sentenced to just one- and two-year sentences.[5]

Some will know the story of Kalief Browder, but many more will not. His arrest, detention, and death reflect the deep racial disparities in the criminal justice system. His case caught the attention of many in New York City, was repeatedly featured in the *New Yorker*, and was referenced by both President Obama and Supreme Court Justice Anthony Kennedy. More recently, Jay-Z produced a documentary on Kalief's life, and numerous other films and series have featured his story. His tragedy also drew attention to the practice of placing 16- and 17-year-olds in adult jails and in solitary confinement. While the disproportionate rates of arrest and incarceration among young men of color like Kalief Browder are well documented, the brutality of other experiences that harm their health behind bars is less well known. There is no reason to believe that the racial disparities that steer greater shares of black and Latino youth toward incarceration wouldn't persist once they arrive there. But the paramilitary nature of jails and prisons shuns transparency, and correctional management is rarely based on rational analysis of data. As we examined our own health service at Rikers, where Kalief Browder was held, we found disturbing evidence that white patients were more likely to receive mental health treatment while in jail, while nonwhite patients were more prone to be punished with solitary confinement.

At the core of these jail-based disparities is a hidden punishment apparatus that propels more than twice as many blacks as whites into solitary confinement. Every jail and prison has a set of rules for people held there, and in the United States, the official consequences for being found guilty of breaking these rules can be anything from a verbal warning, to loss of privileges, to sentences of solitary confinement. It's also important to note that patients routinely report to us that the infraction process is used as a way to keep inmates quiet about abuse. At infraction "hearings" there is no offer of representation and no external oversight. In virtually every instance, when someone is charged with an infraction, the staff bringing the charge, judging the merits of the charge, and hearing the appeal all work for the same group, DOC or the sheriff. The lack of transparency in this process, combined with the deep racial preconceptions baked into criminal justice and health systems, results in a tremendously harmful widening of disparities after people arrive in jail or prison.

For Kalief Browder, his walk home from a party would propel him into a brutal jail setting, where he was subjected to the physical violence of other inmates and correction officers and the mental trauma of solitary confinement. When the case against him finally evaporated after three years, he left Rikers Island as a battered young man. After making progress by starting college and advocating against solitary confinement, the torment of Kalief Browder's three years in jail proved too great a burden, and he took his own life.

For Kalief Browder, 16 years old and a first-time resident in RNDC, his sole priority was likely survival. As he related in the *New Yorker*, "The dayroom was ruled over by a gang leader and his friends, who controlled inmates' access to the prison phones and dictated who could sit on a bench to watch TV and who had to sit on the floor. 'A lot of times, I'd say, "I'm not sitting on the floor," ' Browder said. 'And then they'll come with five or six dudes. They'd swing on me. I'd have to fight back.'" For Kalief, the beatings were not only at the hands of other inmates. He reported that correction officers beat him and other inmates and threatened them with infractions and solitary confinement if they reported their injuries to medical staff. Several years later, it would become clear that using threats to keep injuries hidden was not a problem limited to individual correction officers, but a systemic problem.[6]

KALIEF BROWDER'S TRAGIC EXPERIENCE has helped to galvanize national attention on the racial disparities in our criminal justice system. We had long wondered about racial disparities in our own health service, but even with our electronic medical record, we suspected that the relatively low number of white patients in jail would make an analysis difficult. I reached out to colleagues who helped me understand how important it was to look at this part of our service. Kathy Boudin and Five Mualimm-ak were national experts on criminal justice and had both experienced solitary confinement. They became regular contributors to our human rights meetings and shared their views of the basic unfairness in how prison and jail rules were applied. At a meeting with the American Civil Liberties Union (ACLU), another mentor and national expert on solitary confinement, Dr. Craig Haney, recounted similar observations. He told me that he was quite certain that nonwhite patients were more often victimized by the infraction process. All three of these intelligent colleagues reinforced the degree to which the mental health service is entangled with the punishment apparatus. They shared stories and ideas about how many people end up in the mental health service as a result of spending time in solitary confinement.

So although we knew that it would be hard, we designed an analysis to assess race- and age-related disparities in the entry to the mental health system, as well as the exposure to solitary confinement. We focused on first-time jail admissions, with 45,189 cases occurring between 2011 and 2013.[7] First-time admissions would let us home in on the way in which the jail system first responds to people, which labels were applied, and how the decisions about treatment and punishment were made. Among our cohort, about 41 percent were Latino, 46 percent black, 9 percent white, and 4 percent other. We looked at who came into the mental health service, who went into solitary confinement, and when these two variables occurred together. We also looked at diagnoses, knowing that some jail diagnoses are viewed as more legitimate than others. For example, being diagnosed with depression, schizophrenia, anxiety, or bipolar disorder was often viewed by security and health staff alike as more "legitimate," while people diagnosed with personality disorders, especially antisocial personality disorder, were often viewed as problematic or not really being sick.

What we found when we looked at the mental health service surprised us. Half as many black and Latino patients (as compared to whites) ever entered the mental health service, even when we adjusted for length of stay. Remember that this is despite white inmates being just 9 percent of the population. Most patients enter the mental health service during their first days in jail, either because they report concerns to our health staff or following our review of their records during the intake process. So this disparity might reflect levels of mental health care access in the community, where fewer nonwhite patients engage in mental health care.[8]

Next, we looked at who went into solitary during their stay. Black and Latino patients were much more likely to enter solitary confinement than whites. When we adjusted for length of stay, the likelihood that black patients ever entered solitary was 2.52 times greater than that for whites. For Latino patients, the risk of solitary was 1.88 times greater than that for whites. While many have documented the disparities in arrests and convictions in the United States, this is the first large-scale analysis to report disproportionate application of solitary confinement to nonwhites. It was clear that we had a huge racial imbalance, both in who was sent to solitary and in who received mental health care. If we were to dig deeper, would we find the mechanisms that lead to these differences?

We continued, looking for some interplay between the decisions to treat and to punish, specifically regarding *when* people came into the mental health service. This is critical because early entry into mental health service usually occurs because the patient and/or their jail health providers have identified a clinical issue. We observed that patients who came into the mental health service early in their stay were more likely to be designated as seriously mentally ill, an important indicator that informs jail and discharge planning. We also saw that those who entered the mental health service in the first week were more likely to receive diagnoses of depression and anxiety, while those who came into the services later were more likely to receive diagnoses of mood, antisocial, or adjustment disorder. Patients who enter the mental health service later in their stay often do so because of solitary confinement. Many patients sentenced to solitary hurt themselves in attempts to escape the inhumane punishment. Could a link between those disparities show us the root of the problem?

To find out, we looked at the subset of patients who entered the jail mental health service and whether or not they experienced solitary. Patients with no solitary during jail entered the mental health service in the first days of jail, with 70 percent entering by day 7, and trailing off steadily as time went on. For patients who both experienced solitary and entered the mental health service, we saw a different pattern. Entry into the mental health service was instead neatly grouped around the day they entered solitary, and only 35 percent of them entered the mental health service in their first week of jail. For these patients, entry to the mental health service and solitary confinement appeared to be linked, suggesting that solitary was the key event that would predict whether someone who wasn't already in mental health care soon would be. When we assessed the racial breakdown of these groupings, among those who came into the mental health service later than day 7, only 9 percent of the white patients went into solitary, while 39 percent of black and 26 percent of Latino patients did. Taken together, this shows that nonwhite people are more likely to receive punishment than treatment in jail, whereas whites are not only more likely to receive treatment but also more likely to receive treatment in a true clinical (nonpunishment) context. The obvious link between solitary and patients entering mental health services makes the questions around the entry into solitary, and the practice as a whole, all the more urgent.

There are a couple of possible explanations for what we saw in the solitary-linked mental health encounters. One is that nonwhite patients may not be engaged in care before they enter the jails and their symptoms later on reflect undiagnosed mental illness. Some of this surely happens, but another view, which tracks with my own experience in caring for these patients, is that these symptoms of distress and acts of self-harm reflect normal human reactions to the stress of solitary confinement.

Time after time I've heard from patients that they ended up in solitary because they had to fight when challenged in their housing area, or for other reasons completely unrelated to maintaining the security of the jails. Once in solitary, they felt the stress and pain of the setting, often leading to a cascade of behavioral problems and repeated infractions. Medicalizing these normal human reactions along racial lines has a historical precedent. In the 1850s, American physician Samuel Cartwright coined the term "drapetomania," which he claimed was a psychological disease that caused slaves to flee captivity. In his work "Diseases and Peculiarities of the Negro Race," he wrote, "If any one or more of them, at any time, are inclined to raise their heads to a level with their master or overseer, humanity and their own good requires that they should be punished until they fall into that submissive state which was intended for them to occupy. They have only to be kept in that state, and treated like children to prevent and cure them from running away."[9] It makes my skin crawl to think of a medical doctor inventing a disease to justify both slavery and the abuse that he recommended as treatment. And looking at our solitary population, mostly black and Latino, it seems possible that we're doing the same thing again.

Kalief Browder's rocky introduction to Rikers quickly resulted in him receiving infractions and being sent to solitary confinement. He was held in the central punitive segregation unit, known by everyone on Rikers as "the Bing." Amid the decay of the aging jails on Rikers Island, the Bing was a sturdy, new five-story building dedicated to solitary confinement. One of the first things I would show visitors to Rikers during this period was the Bing and another solitary unit, also new and imposing. They reminded me of the buildings that Joseph Stalin had placed in Eastern European cities to ensure that nobody ever forgot where power sat.

In the Bing, Kalief suffered through intense heat, the chaos of constant yelling, violence, and the mind-numbing boredom of having nothing to do. While it may seem illogical that fights occur on solitary units, where people are held in their cells almost all the time, my experience was that fights and assaults in these areas, including both staff and inmates, were routine. I also came to appreciate that even the highest level of security could be overcome when violence was planned ahead of time. I once found myself in a blood-soaked elevator responding to a near-fatal slashing, and as one part of my brain processed the clinical issues, another wondered how the incident was possible, because both the victim and aggressor had special security status that mandated multiple officers and waist chain restraints at all times. On a solitary unit, the transfer of inmates to showers, recreation, medical visits, and other appointments meant that more than one person was often moving across the tier. Add in the abuse by security staff, which would often include directed beatings and staged fights with inmates, and these units were extremely chaotic. For Kalief Browder, his first stint in solitary lasted two weeks, followed by several others for longer periods. Eventually, he would be placed in solitary for 10 months and then even longer. Amid the chaos and depersonalization of solitary, there are daily challenges that can be difficult to navigate. Every inmate is supposed to be offered a daily shower and an hour of recreation time, but many people don't go to rec, either because it isn't truly offered or because of the stress and vulnerability of standing, placing one's hands backward out the food slot in the cell door to be rear-cuffed, and then being escorted to a small cage the size of a dog kennel for an hour.[10]

Kalief also reported a type of DOC assault that I had long heard about but almost couldn't believe until I saw it with my own eyes a couple of years later. He told Jennifer Gonnerman of the *New Yorker* that an officer took offense at something he said and then challenged him to a fight. The officer came to his cell to fight, but not alone; Kalief was jumped by multiple officers and beaten. The cases I came to know about would sometimes look exactly like a schoolyard fight, with officers taking off their pepper spray, badge, and other gear and then having a fight with an inmate. Eventually, the violence and stress took its toll on Kalief Browder. In February 2012, over 600 days into his incarceration, he ripped up his sheets inside his solitary cell, tied them into a rope, and tried to hang himself. Guards saw him attempting to hang himself and took him to the jail health clinic. But ultimately he was put right back in solitary.

The decision to offer a treatment or punishment response to problems in jail has a profound and lasting impact on the millions of people who pass through jails and prisons every year. We strayed into this topic during discussions of traumatic brain injury (TBI) with adolescent patients in 2012.[11] We had discovered through screenings that half of adolescents in jail had a history of TBI.[12] Exploring the circumstances that lead to TBI in focus groups, we quickly learned that survival in the jails was a violent enterprise. While anyone would rather not suffer a blow to the head, there were much higher priorities that often made it impossible to avoid for most.

We began each conversation with a short video clip that depicted a violent blow to the head. The facilitator then asked a series of open-ended questions, including "What is your reaction to the violence in the clips you just watched?" and "How does violence in jail compare to violence in the community?" Each focus group started with these broad questions but inevitably turned to questions of power, race, and inequity, especially in the jails. One participant stated, "The tough thing is, when we fight someone, we're doing it to actually hurt them . . . we want them to make sure they are in pain for what they did to us." Another participant described how you "feel like you have to be a bigger man by hurting the next man." Each focus group then split into smaller groups, with the adolescents developing their own grouping of causes and consequences of violence, relating to personal, community, and societal factors.

The results from these groups revealed how race impacts the experiences of people in jail. It was striking to us in the health service that our patients treated the racial differences in their exposure to jail violence as matter-of-fact. This disconnect is part of the hypocrisy of American incarceration: the incarcerated endure inconsistent, violent, and biased treatment, while those who run the jails and prisons and the community at large act as if it's the inmates who create strife and discord. Common themes from our focus groups included the role of racial and income disparities in violence, the use of violence as capital, and the inevitability of violence. Many participants discussed the need for violence as a basic survival tool in jail. One adolescent reported, "A short-term show of violence can scare off more serious violence later." Another stated, "Reputations are like currency in jail. Your reputation can determine whether you get an extra tray of food in the box or a nice cut at the barber shop." Some discussed the impossibility of avoiding this dynamic in jail. Said one, "There is no place to go [without] someone bother[ing] you . . . in jail you see a lot of crazy shit. Correctional officers punching inmates, stabbings, knives in cells; I've seen one guy use a scalpel. [They make] weapons out of anything, like toilet pieces." Some respondents acknowledged that correction officers were trapped in the same dynamic: "If he puts his hands on someone that generates respect in the house." Others identified the need for alternative approaches: "It's important to talk to people you respect who are going through the same thing. You can lessen the pain by speaking to each other."

Kalief fought in order to avoid more fights. And when he couldn't escape the need to fight, it chipped away at his spirit. If his experiences in jail were characterized by brutality, his treatment by the legal system was marked by indifference and incompetence. Kalief's case was relatively straightforward: one person claimed that Kalief and his friend had assaulted him and robbed him of a backpack containing electronics and cash. But time after time, the prosecutors, defense, and judge in Kalief's case would not be ready or available for key hearings and trial dates. Throughout his stays in solitary, Kalief refused to take a plea in his case, insisting on his innocence.

Inside the jails, there is plenty of advice on how to handle one's case, and young detainees are often emboldened to stick it out through trial in the hopes that the case against them will fall apart or that they will get a favorable deal. At the same time, prosecutors rely on the horrors of Rikers to coerce defendants into accepting a plea deal.

Families are profoundly influenced by the coercive power of Rikers as well. The visitation process is humiliating and anxiety producing and involves many hours of transport and waiting while hoping for a short visit. For families that cannot make bail for their loved ones, the prospect of a plea deal can be welcome news. It would mean a release from the danger and indignity of Rikers. Almost lost in this struggle between survival and dominance is the idea that any defendant in Rikers who pleads guilty may be innocent of the charges against them.

But despite (or maybe in defiance of) the horrors he suffered, Kalief Browder did not leap at the chance for a plea deal. On the 74th day of his detention, he was indicted and pleaded not guilty. In early 2012, about two years and eight months into his detention, Kalief turned down another plea offer of three and a half years, despite facing a potential of 15 years if found guilty at trial. In March 2013, Kalief went to court and met the eighth judge involved in his case. As part of an effort to reduce the backlogs of court cases in the Bronx, this judge offered Kalief a deal: admit guilt to two misdemeanor charges with a 16-month sentence, essentially time served thus far. This deal would have allowed him to go home that day. Kalief refused, insisting that he was innocent, and was returned to Rikers, where he stayed until another court appearance in May 2013. This time, the judge had shocking news. The complainant against Kalief could no longer be located, and thus the case was being dismissed. Kalief spent one more night in RNDC as paperwork was completed, and then he was released the next day. He had entered Rikers as a 16-year-old; he returned home to his mother a few days after his 20th birthday.

Back at home, Kalief found himself acting withdrawn and avoiding many of the social settings and experiences that he had enjoyed before Rikers. As he told Jennifer Gonnerman, "I'm trying to break out of my shell, but I guess there is no shell. I guess this is just how I am—I'm just quiet and distant," he says. "I don't like being this way, but it's just natural to me now." Kalief worked to get his life back on track. He had missed his junior and senior years of high school, and although there was supposed to be some education available during his time in solitary, it really amounted to officers randomly dropping off and picking up worksheets, with rare visits from teachers. In the months after being released from Rikers, Kalief initiated a lawsuit against NYC for his incarceration and treatment. But his struggle with depression that had begun in jail persisted, and Kalief attempted suicide six months after his release, trying to hang himself in November 2013, just as he had a year and a half earlier in solitary confinement.

After an inpatient psychiatric hospitalization, Kalief returned home. He made progress on his goals, earning his GED and starting classes at Bronx Community College. His case seemed to build momentum; celebrities and politicians cited it as an example of the deep problems with the criminal justice system. Months after his release, Jennifer Gonnerman obtained video from Rikers of Kalief being assaulted by correction officers. He insisted on sharing that video on the *New Yorker* website, just as he had insisted on his own innocence. He wrote an essay in his Bronx Community College courses about the harms of solitary confinement. Kalief was free. People were on his side, and to say that Kalief was a young man of uncommon strength of will would be an understatement. But despite all of his determination, Kalief could not overcome the enduring pain Rikers had inflicted. On June 6, 2014, he ripped his bed sheets into strips, as he had done in Rikers, and hanged himself from his window frame at home. His mother, who had called him "peanut" from childhood, heard the thump of his body weight hitting the window frame and rushed outside to find him hanging.[13]

Kalief Browder's story caught the attention of people across the globe because of the tragedy and injustice he suffered, but his was only one of the roughly 12 million incarcerations that occur each year in the United

States. These incarcerations leave their mark on everyone who heads home or moves from jail to prison, and the health consequences may be hard to define. For Kalief Browder, his struggles with depression and depersonalization may have also been exacerbated by physical trauma.

One of the outgrowths of our work on TBI was to think about how violence in jail might create long-term public health crises for communities with high incarceration rates. Almost all of the 12 million annual arrests result in a return home, and the impact of physical and emotional trauma lasts well beyond the time one is locked up. To assess how hidden head trauma in jail is, we looked at the amount of jail-based head trauma (and the subset that meets criteria for TBI) that results in patient transfer to the hospital. Hospital transfer is important for individual patients, but it's also important for us as a society to know about, because only through contact with a community health provider can the Centers for Disease Control and Prevention and other public health agencies track head trauma. As we've seen, jails don't report injuries. In the past few years, football players and their fans and families have heard quite a bit about the link between TBI and chronic traumatic encephalopathy (CTE), a syndrome of behavioral changes linked to prior head trauma. Although understanding of the mechanism of CTE is still evolving, we believe that repeated head trauma causes changes in the brain years later that can drive extreme behaviors. These behaviors range from aggression and violence to social withdrawal and suicide. The characteristic scarring of brain tissue that is associated with CTE has been present in the brains of several National Football League players who have committed suicide, including Junior Seau, Andre Waters, and Dave Duerson. All of our national discussion about CTE has related to contact sports, particularly football. Some attention has been given recently to the prevalence of TBI and CTE in military personnel, but there has been no discussion of the rates of TBI in jail or the potential consequences down the road for those who, like Kalief Browder, return home after experiencing violence. Our review of TBI in Rikers over 42 months found about 10,000 instances of head trauma and 1,500 cases of TBI. These rates are about 50 times higher than what is reported in the community for all causes, with 14 and 55 percent of these cases, respectively, resulting in hospital transfer.[14] When we converted these rates to estimates of the entire American jail/prison population, we projected that each year in the United States there are about

600,000 head injuries in correctional settings and 90,000 cases of TBI. Applying our hospitalization rates nationally, about 500,000 patients with head injuries and 40,000 patients with TBI are not transferred to the hospital. Consequently, all of those patients are off the radar of our national health surveillance for downstream effects like CTE. The short-term physical and emotional toll of these incidents is daunting, but the long-term implications for CTE prevalence in communities disproportionately impacted by mass incarceration are horrifying.

THE EXPERIENCES OF KALIEF BROWDER were not an unfortunate turn of events. They were a man-made disaster. Many would view his release and lawsuit against NYC as a correction of a wrong. When he spoke of his experiences to the *New Yorker*, he summed it up like this: "People tell me because I have this case against the city I'm all right. But I'm not all right. I'm messed up. I know that I might see some money from this case, but that's not going to help me mentally. I'm mentally scarred right now. That's how I feel. Because there are certain things that changed about me and they might not go back." His story, as well as our data, tells us that the health consequences of incarceration are distributed along racial lines. This is not a shock to anyone who knows the criminal justice system. They know how interwoven the health and security systems are inside jails in deciding who merits treatment and who should be punished. One of the central hypocrisies of mass incarceration is to fail at basic management and then punish the incarcerated for these failures. The widespread use of violence as a basic tool of control by security staff forces the incarcerated to trade in the same currency. The lack of connection between the rules and reality leads naturally to the security authority selectively enforcing their rules. Like other settings where transparency and accountability are in short supply, selective enforcement breaks along racial lines.[15]

The revelation that we provide care in the same racially divided way that the security service enforces their rules is both distressing and predictable. We know that significant disparities exist in the mental health services provided outside jail, so patients arrive with these accumulated differences.[16] Others before us have also identified racial disparities in mental health diagnoses in correctional settings, whether by self-report or by clinical diagnosis.[17] Doctors, nurses, social workers—we can all be susceptible to the same preconceptions about race and punishment as the corrections officers. And whether the health staff start out with these preconceptions or not, bias is baked into the processes around solitary. Because most jails and prisons require health staff to "clear" people for solitary confinement, the inequities in the punishment apparatus are presented to health staff every time someone is punished with solitary confinement. The consequences exist on both sides of the patient/provider relationship. We can see the damage that this clearance process does, as patients quickly come to see us as part of the punishment system. Health and security systems are at the heart of widening racial disparities in jail. The infraction process operates as an unaccountable system of rules enforcement that doles out solitary confinement along racial lines. Detainees have no right to representation in this process, and they often incur both new financial penalties and punishment as a result of infractions. Depending on the jail system, these infractions may stay on the books forever, so that each entry to jail brings a return to solitary confinement, even for a long-distant rules violation. There is no transparency in the infraction process, and no expectation of fair treatment. I question its stated purpose: to deliver swift consequences for rules violations and thereby promote security. Solitary doesn't discourage violence. Dr. Robert Morris of the University of Texas analyzed data from 70 prisons and found that among inmates who received solitary confinement for violent infractions, solitary had no impact on the likelihood of subsequent violent infractions.[18] The experiences of Kalief Browder and others also reveal the link between solitary confinement and violence by security staff.

As with the other health risks of incarceration, those driven by race can be addressed. First of all, health staff in jails and prisons should be trained on the racial disparities inherent in their system and the potential for their work to further widen the racial divide between treatment and punishment. NYC received federal funding to start this type of training with our health staff, and they have responded.[19] However, educating staff doesn't help patients unless it's accompanied by other structural changes. In order for health staff to truly address these concerns, we must uncouple them from the racist punishment system. Removing health staff from the job of "clearing" people for solitary confinement is important. We need real oversight and accountability in infraction processes. DOCs and sheriffs should be compelled to report data on infractions, and the people subject to these processes should be entitled to representation overseen by external authorities. But even with better training and accountability inside jails and prisons, health consequences will fall along racial lines until the upstream fundamentals of mass incarceration are addressed. Undoing mass incarceration will require active efforts to maintain a commitment to racial fairness throughout the progress that is made. Some settings, like NYC, have made substantial gains in reducing overall rates of incarceration but have been unable to make real changes to the disproportionately black and Latino demographics of the incarcerated.

The necessary work involves far more than sentencing reform, however. The interminable delays that Kalief Browder experienced reflect deep problems in the district attorney's office, as well as the lack of resources in the public defense and court systems. These shortcomings disproportionately impact the poor and people of color across the United States. In Louisiana, the ACLU has reported that people who need a public defender are being incarcerated without ever seeing a lawyer.[20] Despite the numerous constitutional and other legal principles that seemingly guarantee the right to counsel in the United States, practices in Louisiana reflect the collision between the nation's highest rates of incarceration and complete dismantling of public defense and other elementary safeguards against the criminal justice system. The losers in Louisiana, as with most of the other mismatched struggles between the need to incarcerate and the promise of justice and fairness, are mostly people of color like Kalief Browder.

It's important to remember that Kalief Browder did not succumb to his fate out of weakness. He was not a willing or indifferent victim. He railed and resisted the system that beat him down, and when he had the opportunity to escape its clutches with an admission of guilt, he refused. He fought every attempt to coerce a guilty plea from him, even as his spirit and body suffered the consequences. Once free of Rikers, he turned his attention to furthering his own education, and he spread the word of the brutality and unfairness of incarceration to millions through speaking and television appearances.

Similar were the struggles of other young men profiled in this book who died at Rikers: Christopher Robinson, Jason Echevarria, Angel Ramirez, Bradley Ballard, and Carlos Mercado. All of these patients suffered because the jail system met their problems with punishment rather than treatment. All of these patients died unnecessarily, as a clear consequence of incarceration, and not one of them was white. These deaths generated many press stories and ample outrage, but efforts on their behalf should push us to do more than look for bad apples or individual errors. We should reconsider the risks and benefits of incarceration in the United States and maintain a focus on promoting racial fairness in each of the reform efforts we undertake.

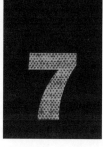

Sexual Assault in Rikers

Maria and Brianna

THE SEXUAL ABUSE OF MARIA started when a correction officer assigned to her housing area began to monitor her while she worked on the daytime cleaning detail and the other housing area officer slept. It was about a week after she arrived in jail, and the officer, one of those regularly assigned to her housing area, made Maria feel uncomfortable with his staring at her. A pattern quickly developed during this officer's regular shifts. He would give her orders to clean various parts of the housing area and then ogle her as she completed her work. This "work" was often given to Maria early in the morning, while others slept, and was accompanied by unsolicited comments from the officer about his personal life, including his relationship with his wife. One day, the officer exposed himself to Maria, and she felt too terrified to walk away. A week later, after another similar incident, Maria did try to walk away, at which time the officer said that he wanted Maria "to be his" and ordered that she come to an unoccupied room in the evening, when he would work an extra shift. That is when he raped Maria, and he went on to assault her on a regular basis. During these assaults, the officer would often choke Maria and threaten her to ensure her silence. These assaults were apparently made possible because the supervisory staff (captains) were often not at their posts and many correction officers slept during their shifts. Aside from being on a cleaning detail that involved some movement from one area to another, Maria was also likely an attractive victim because of her intellectual disability. Working in the jails has taught me many lessons about the patterns of predators. Every new arrival to a housing area is closely scanned by the other patients, as well as by the correctional officers. For those with malicious intent, careful attention will be paid to how isolated, confused, or anxious someone is. These characteristics provide openings for abuse in many forms, from extorting someone for protection to giving them preferable treatment as a setup for sexual abuse. Maria had been a special education student in school and was held back twice before she dropped out of 10th grade. When she left school, she had tested in the bottom 0.5 percent of her group for verbal comprehension, a ripe target for abuse in the complex and violent jail setting.

Few will be surprised that sexual assault is a significant health risk of incarceration. Rape and other forms of sexual abuse permeate most cultural references about going to jail or prison. Culturally we have come to accept sexual assault behind bars so completely that it has become a punch line to discussions about incarceration. This chapter focuses on the reported sexual abuse of two women who are part of a class action lawsuit against New York City.[1] The lawsuit makes the claim that sexual abuse of inmates is widespread, common knowledge, and essentially accepted by corrections officials and includes the reports of abuse of Maria and Brianna. The abuse documented in this lawsuit started in 2008, about the same time that an extremely important federal law, the Prison Rape Elimination Act (PREA), was coming into effect in American prisons and jails. PREA represents the only area of health risks of incarceration where all jails and prisons are supposed to follow a uniform approach to surveillance, case response, reporting, and mitigation. PREA was first implemented in state prison systems and more recently adopted in local jails. Because jails usually receive little federal funding, the potential punishment for noncompliance is relatively small, and some systems, like NYC, have been slow to adopt the principles. Our own efforts in correctional health to document sexual abuse started around the time of Maria's and Brianna's abuse. Our early meetings with security officials about this topic yielded a confounding but resolute refusal to acknowledge the scope or severity of the problem. However, once press coverage of Rikers exploded in 2014, the long-standing problem of sexual assault became an important part of the Rikers discussion for those in oversight of the jails if not the security service itself.

By 2015, the coverage of the Bradley Ballard and Jerome Murdough deaths, together with Kalief Browder's case and the US Department of Justice investigation, had resulted in almost daily press stories about abuse and neglect at Rikers. Local authorities in NYC, including the Public Advocate, began to push the Department of Correction to collect and reveal more information about sexual abuse in the jails, an effort that was long overdue. In April of 2015 the oversight body of the jails, the Board of Correction, exerted its authority. Despite PREA being a federal law, the Board of Correction and others understood that creating a local law with similar focus would help them to enforce these mandates in the NYC jails more effectively. The arduous process of designing and approving the Board of Correction PREA rule took almost 18 months, but by November 2016 PREA was in effect on Rikers Island.

One of the core assumptions of PREA, and of this book, is that abuse reflects failures of institutions, not just the actions of a few bad apples. Jails and prisons are often designed and run in a manner that avoids transparency or accountability. This enables staff to attack and belittle those who suffer abuse and those who would dare report it. The sexual abuse of Maria, Brianna, and countless others is one of the many ways in which these systems are responsible for damaging the health of the incarcerated.

Jail is a rich hunting ground. I can't overstate the ease with which sexual predators can observe potential victims, plan their abuse, and leverage the jail to retaliate against victims and ensure their silence. When these women reported that they were abused by the same correction officer over many years and incarcerations, and with the apparent knowledge and complicity of other officers, it led to a class action lawsuit against NYC. A core assertion of the suit is that sexual abuse at Rikers is commonplace and that there are many other victims and perpetrators. This assertion is strongly supported by data collected by us in the correctional health service, as well as by the DOJ. For both Maria and Brianna, victimization involved a correctional officer deftly leveraging their personal vulnerabilities into points of control and violence.

Once the officer established control of Maria, he sexually assaulted her regularly, up to four times per week, whenever she was in jail. Maria was released from Rikers, but when she returned in 2011, the same officer was still working there and was angry with her for not visiting him at his home, as she had been ordered to do when she last left. The physical, emotional, and sexual abuse of Maria restarted almost as soon as she arrived back in jail. The officer sometimes instructed her to report chest pains, so that she would be escorted to the medical clinic. Once there, she was told to say that the pains had resolved, creating an opportunity for the officer to escort Maria back to her housing area. Because the officer had keys to unused parts of the jail, and because of the lack of supervision, he could easily take Maria to those places and assault her along the way. This incarceration lasted over a year, with constant assaults and threats from this officer against Maria.

During this period of abuse of Maria, we in correctional health were just beginning to track and report all types of injury in the NYC jails, including sexual abuse. PREA was not yet considered to be in effect by NYC, and many of our efforts occurred in a vacuum. Although very few patients were reporting sexual abuse to us at this time, the DOJ was conducting phone surveys of detainees, and almost 9 percent of women reported being sexually abused, the highest rate in the nation, about three times higher than the national average.[2] As we improved our own reporting and care in correctional health, the number of patients who felt safe telling us about sexual abuse steadily increased. By 2014, we developed comprehensive reports to show the nature of sexual abuse and the profiles of the patients and their jail setting. In 2015, we received about 10–15 complaints per month, with roughly half of the reports made against correctional officers. We also saw that women, people in the mental health service, and LGBTQ (lesbian, gay, bisexual, transgender, and queer) patients were far more likely to report sexual abuse, consistent with the observations of the DOJ.[3]

The sexual abuse of Brianna also followed the patterns of observation, stalking, and abuse. Brianna encountered the correction officer in question in 2013, when she was incarcerated on Rikers and doing the job of suicide prevention aid. This position was one of the more coveted inmate jobs and involved training on recognition of the signs of suicidality among inmates and moving throughout housing areas to monitor other inmates and refer them to the mental health service when they seemed to be struggling. Several days after an innocuous encounter with an officer while Brianna was performing her suicide prevention duties, he stopped her, made lewd comments to her, and offered to pay her for oral sex. A short time later, the officer found Brianna and asked her not to report his behavior, which she agreed to. Several days later, Brianna was instructed by this officer to leave her suicide prevention duties and meet him in the pantry after captains had made their rounds of the jail. When she arrived, the officer gave her some contraband items and took her to an area off camera, the janitor's slop sink closet, where he forced her to perform oral sex. Afterward he gave her a bible study book with his personal information written inside. Almost every night that the officer was on duty, he would instruct Brianna to meet him in the pantry area, where he would rape her. The officer also instructed Brianna to request switching her suicide prevention shift to better match his work schedule. During this time, Brianna was almost never able to complete her suicide prevention rounds, which are supposed to be done every 15 minutes. Her absence from her designated work site and her inability to completely document her work endangered other inmates and was obvious to multiple officers. At one point, one of the officers told Brianna, "What you're doing isn't right," but nobody stood up for her or other victims to stop the abuse.

For both Maria and Brianna, there would come a time when their abuser would use violence, threats, and complicity of other officers to ensure their silence. Sexual abuse often involves shaming and violence to ensure compliance, but in jail there is such a profound power imbalance between detainees and correction officers that the threats made against the abused are very credible and their recourse extremely limited. In the case of Maria, there came a time when she refused sexual contact with the correction officer, which he responded to by anally raping her. He did the same when he saw her make eye contact with other correctional officers. On more than one instance, Maria asked the officer to use a condom, and his "punishment" of her would be the same.

Another aspect of this subjugation was to force Maria to involve her family as victims. The officer forced Maria to give the officer contact information for her mother. The officer would give small amounts of money to Maria's mother to put into her jail commissary account, establishing dominance over her life outside jail as well as on the inside. At one point, the officer told Maria that she would have to live with him when she left jail. The threats against Maria's family were real and comprehensive. The officer told her that he had visited her mothers' house on multiple occasions, sometimes introducing himself as a "friend" and other times sitting in his car watching her family, including small nieces. The access of correctional officers to family members of the incarcerated can be a powerful tool of control, humiliation, or threat. One Friday evening I went to see an agitated patient who had suffered serious injury from a use of force that occurred during a visit with a loved one. He said that a misunderstanding with guards resulted in them taking him to an area off camera and beating him severely. His worry had nothing to do with his own injuries, though. He was worried sick because his loved one had reportedly been followed off Rikers by one of the guards who had beaten him, stopped, and forced to give over her personal information. The ability of his abusers to contact his family members was a far more agonizing experience for this man than being beaten.

For Brianna, the efforts to humiliate and control her were even more wide-ranging than those suffered by Maria. After receiving contraband items from the correctional officer who was sexually abusing her, Brianna was caught with these items by other officers and subjected to 15 days of solitary confinement. Despite never saying where she received the contraband, Brianna was then subject to a campaign of abuse from other inmates, orchestrated by the officer who was abusing her and who thought she had reported him. He, or other officers, let some detainees out of their cells at night, when everyone was supposed to be locked in. The detainees would then congregate around Brianna's cell door and yell threats at her. This tactic of control, selective opening of other inmates' cell doors, was used by correctional officers in the beating death of 18-year-old Christopher Robinson in 2008 (see chap. 2). In addition, the officers working in Brianna's housing area would refuse to let her out for showers or recreation and would withhold her food. This abuse created such emotional strain that Brianna told one of the officers that she wanted to take her own life. The officer opened her cell door, only to have a group of detainees encircle Brianna, screaming that they would kill her. When she was finally taken to see mental health staff, Brianna reported the abuse she had been experiencing, and the health staffer contacted the Department of Investigation.

According to the lawsuit, Brianna was transferred to another housing area once she reported the sexual abuse, but a new campaign of harassment and abuse was initiated by officers there, who were angered that she had reported their colleague. She was told that she was "wrong" for reporting the abuse and called a "snitch," "bitch," or "famous" often by groups of officers who would congregate outside her cell door. After some time, Brianna was transferred to another jail for her protection, but eventually she returned to Rikers because of her court case. Upon her return, she was placed in solitary confinement for no apparent reason, and the group harassment by officers started back up. Legal Aid began to advocate on behalf of Brianna, but at some point a captain forced her to sign a document stating that she had never been harassed by any Rikers correction officer. Although she signed this forced confession out of fear, she mustered one small act of resistance by signing someone else's name. This type of intimidation against reporting was also documented by the DOJ in their investigation of brutality against adolescents. In one instance, "an inmate stated that when he asked staff for medical attention after being raped by an officer, he was told not to say anything about the incident. He reported it anyway, and told our consultant that after doing so, staff continually harassed him. In fact, the inmate reported to our consultant that he was warned by two officers not to say anything about the incident as he was being taken to speak with our consultant while our investigative team was at Rikers."[4] This account reveals an especially brazen culture, where staff feel emboldened not only to discourage victims from seeking care or reporting abuse through intimidation but also to interfere with DOJ investigations. As if the many ordeals were not enough, Brianna was told when she arrived at the state prison system that she had contracted a sexually transmitted infection.

In medicine, we use the term "nosocomial" to describe infections that originate from the hospital setting itself. A patient may be hospitalized as a result of a horrible car wreck, but the infection they get while on a breathing machine is considered nosocomial. Much the same can be said of sexual abuse behind bars, but whereas a hospital patient who takes an unexpected turn for the worse sets off alarms both real and metaphorical, triggering a flurry of activity, there is not much outcry when the incarcerated are sexually abused. The original congressional hearings for PREA included horrific testimony by formerly incarcerated people who described how their sexual abuse was not only tolerated but also sometimes supported or directed by correctional staff. I've taken to thinking of this as *nosocomial rape*—a condition caused by the setting. One of the stories that galvanized bipartisan support for PREA was that of Rodney Hulin, a 17-year-old, 126-pound adolescent incarcerated in Texas. His father testified,

My name is Rodney Hulin and I work at a retirement home here in Beaumont, Texas. I am here today because of my son. He would be here himself if he could. . . . But he can't because he died. . . . My son was raped and sodomized by an inmate. The doctor found two tears in his rectum and ordered an HIV test, since up to a third of the 2,200 inmates there were HIV positive. Fearing for his safety, he requested to be placed in protective custody, but his request was denied because, as the warden put it, "Rodney's abuses didn't meet the 'emergency grievance criteria.'" For the next several months, my son was repeatedly beaten by the older inmates, forced to perform oral sex, robbed, and beaten again. Each time, his requests for protection were denied by the warden. The abuses, meanwhile, continued. On the night of January 26, 1996—seventy-five days after my son entered Clemens—Rodney attempted suicide by hanging himself in his cell. He could no longer stand to live in continual terror. It was too much for him to handle. He laid in a coma for the next four months until he died.[5]

One of the most damning aspects of this and numerous other cases is that Rodney Hulin reported his abuse and repeatedly asked for protection. Instead, his abuse continued, and his pleas for protection earned him the label of troublemaker, hardening the security staff against him and emboldening his abusers. In these instances, the role of the institution is not only to permit sexual abuse but also to isolate and retaliate against those who report abuse.

The institutional role in promoting sexual abuse is partly rooted in managerial incompetence of the most basic custodial functions. Early in my time at Rikers, I cared for a patient who escaped from custody by simply wearing a suit to court and waiting for a change of officers in the court pens, at which time he declared himself to be a lawyer and then made his way through a courtroom and out the front door. Having pulled his black socks over his orange shoes, he appeared like any other smartly dressed, white lawyer, and he headed straight from the courthouse to see his mother.[6] Around the same time that Maria was suffering abuse in the women's jail, an ex-inmate was able to use a fake badge to enter multiple jails on Rikers, obtain corrections gear such as a radio and jacket, and have unsupervised contact with detainees, all with the unwitting cooperation of jail managers.

During a series of jail *break-ins* that spanned months, this person report-edly directed that certain inmates be moved from one area to another, where he sexually abused them. As a burly white male, this person raised no alarm bells until he took the incredible step of initiating new criminal charges against detainees for imagined rules violations. When he went to the Bronx courthouse posing as a DOC investigator to press charges against a detainee for a crime committed in jail, his identity was finally questioned, and he was arrested.[7] The ability of an outsider to move throughout the jails unchallenged may seem unreal, but it's a consequence of much more than lax security practices. There has been no shortage of independent report-ing on the dismal state of basic security practices at Rikers, including not using metal detectors for security staff.[8] One of the lessons from reports of sexual abuse in jails is that correctional predators rely on their own ability to move around without any record, just as they also rely on being able to move detainees to more vulnerable or hidden locations. During my time at Rikers, a shadow team of "enforcement" officers was operating in the jails, moving in and out of various jails without signing log books and adminis-tering beatings and interrogations without leaving official record of their presence.[9] Once the brutality of Rikers came into public view, members of this team would be charged and convicted of federal crimes for the assault of Jamal Lightfoot. Taken together, these and many other incidents reflect a system of jails where the movement of detainees and staff was largely unregulated. This ability of staff to move themselves and detainees in an undetected manner is a critical contributor to the sexual abuse suffered by Maria, Brianna, and many others.

But the inability of correctional settings to deal with sexual abuse is not only a matter of lax custodial practices. Security staff often downplay the problem of sexual abuse based on the profile of those who are abused most often (the mentally ill or LGBTQ patients) or because of the litigious nature of incarceration. I will never forget calling a top security official one Sunday to inform him of a sexual abuse allegation, and the first thing he asked me was, "But is it from an MO?" (which was shorthand for a patient with mental illness). To be sure, there are many individual officers, as well as leadership, who see the toll that sexual victimization takes on the incarcerated, and some of these officers often make efforts to help an inmate in ways we might never know. In the horrible case of Rodney Hulin, there was a correction officer, Pablo Salazar, who tried, without success, to help Rodney by advocating that he be granted protective custody. And many a time, my staff and I only came to know about a vulnerable or abused patient because a correctional officer raised the concern to us. But one of the core challenges with sexual abuse of the incarcerated is that correctional officials often view the abuse as being about sex, not about power, control, and violence. Security staff and leadership seem to recognize some of the most egregious cases of sexual abuse as problematic, but because they are enmeshed in the power imbalance between themselves and the incarcerated, they often fail to grasp how sexual abuse and victimization are tools of control. This cultural divide in how we conceptualize sexual abuse is a difficult part of adopting PREA but is at the heart of how correctional settings cause harm when operating normally. Our own data reveal that between one-third and one-half of annual reports of sexual abuse inflicted by security staff indicate that the abuse occurred during a use of force or other "security"-related physical contact. These incidents are often chalked up to sour grapes among detainees who are involved in a use of force with officers and want to retaliate somehow, and they are virtually never substantiated. In 2016, a male detainee reported that hours after a verbal exchange with a correction officer he was called out of his housing area, purportedly to go to the cafeteria. On the way, the captain escorting him was joined by several other officers, and he was slammed up against the wall. He related the following to a reporter: "'He was groping my genitals, grabbing my (expletive), putting his hand between my butt cheeks,' inmate Justin Kuchma said. 'While he's doing all of this, he's asking me if I like it, he's calling me a (expletive). . . . He's kicking me in the shins,' he said. 'As he's done with his search, he pulls my pants down.'"[10] The sexual touching of detainees is a quick and powerful method of humiliation that establishes shame and impotence without causing bruises or broken bones.

One of the most revealing data points during the time in which Maria and Brianna were suffering sexual abuse is the disconnect between anonymous reporting and the number of people who reported abuse to us in the health system. From 2007 to 2013, the annual number of sexual abuse reports steadily increased from 38 to 119. By 2016, we were on track to receive about 400 reports in the year. This is a dramatic increase from prior years, especially given the decrease in the jail population by about 30 percent.

But more concerning is that this number of reports is still far below what we would expect based on the anonymous reports by the DOJ. Based on the DOJ results that 8.6 percent of women and 5.1 percent of men had reported sexual abuse, and allowing for a current rate of 55,000 admissions a year (about 3,500 women), complete sexual abuse reporting would result in about 300 reports among women and 2,600 reports among men in a year. So if we reach 400 reports in 2016, that will be double the prior year but still be about 13 percent of the total we would expect based on the DOJ reports. By comparison, about one-third of rapes are reported to police in the community.[11] We are still a long way from this very modest standard, and while we have done work to improve reporting, there is still clear reluctance among patients to report incidents for fear of retaliation, and the jails appear as chaotic and violent as ever.

THESE STORIES, AND MANY OTHERS, have revealed that investigations into sexual abuse are either nonexistent or incompetent. This shameful neglect is an essential factor that allows rapists to flourish in our jails. At one NYC Board of Correction meeting, a woman gave halting testimony on this topic. She spoke for less than a minute but started by identifying herself as a survivor of sexual assault at Rikers, stating, "I never reported my sexual assault and to this day I have no plans of reporting it. I do not feel comfortable with that and I think that's the way a lot of people feel when they're incarcerated. They don't feel safe."[12] In a three-hour meeting, her one minute of testimony left an indelible impression. The guidelines for conducting investigations into sexual abuse are one of the strongest aspects of PREA, but this woman reflected a valid concern that unfortunately persists in the jails, that reporting sexual abuse makes one a target and the abused are better off remaining quiet.

Letitia James, the NYC Public Advocate, became involved in this issue and joined a group of advocates in pushing the Board of Correction to enact PREA as a set of local rules. One of her first steps was to ask for all the internal reports that we had been compiling in correctional health, and then she compared our sexual abuse numbers from quarter 1 of 2014 and 2015 to DOC numbers on the outcomes of investigations and NYPD data on prosecutions. Over half of the reports of sexual abuse involved accusations of a patient against DOC staff. When we looked at the profiles of patients reporting abuse, several groups stood out. Women constitute about 6 percent of the jail population but accounted for 12 and 15 percent of sexual abuse reports in the six months of reports made public from 2014 and 2015, respectively. Over 90 percent of reports in both quarters came from patients in the mental health service, despite only about two of every five patients in jail being in this cohort. Patients who self-identified as LGBTQ made up nearly half of sexual abuse reports in one of these quarters and almost one of every four in another. Transgender patients, who represent fewer than 1 out of every 10 people in jail, were involved in nearly 3 of every 10 sexual abuse reports. Most damning was that only 2.5 percent of these reports were ever substantiated, and some of those were never referred to NYPD for any action. The annual number of substantiated cases never exceeded 3 in any of these years. If the rate were to match the national average, we would expect 15 of the cases to be proven.[13]

Once public, these data points caused an uproar, much like our use-of-force report or the details of Bradley Ballard's and Jerome Murdough's deaths. The low rate of substantiation is the result of ineffective investigations, not of spurious claims, a truth known by those who would report abuse. City council members, local and state politicians, and advocates in many realms all seized on the numbers as a nearly complete invalidation of reports of sexual abuse victims by DOC. At a New York City Council hearing on this topic in 2016, committee chair Corey Johnson uncovered another contributor to retaliation and intimidation: the lack of any policy about keeping suspected abusers away from their victims. He asked a senior DOC official, "So someone has been accused of potentially raping an individual and they are still allowed to work with inmates while an investigation is going on?"[14] The answer was "yes," and that discretion is given to DOC supervisors to decide for themselves. This exchange fueled even more concern that DOC (and NYC) was not serious about protecting inmates from sexual abuse. NYC has not been alone in resisting the necessary changes. Some states have completely refused to comply with PREA, stating that they have internal measures that are just as effective and less burdensome. In a 2014 letter to the US attorney general, Governor Rick Perry of Texas claimed that Texas would not comply with PREA and touted the success of their internal Safe Prisons Program, including an 84 percent *reduction* in sexual assault reports at juvenile justice facilities.[15] A total of seven states took this stance, among them Governor Mike Pence of Indiana, who argued that compliance with PREA would "require a redirection of millions of tax dollars currently supporting other critical needs for Indiana."[16] Since 2014, most of these states have changed their approach and declared an intent to become PREA compliant, largely because of the threat of lawsuits. In the case of NYC, this process is estimated to take four to five years.

One of the most significant events in NYC was the enactment of a rule by the NYC Board of Correction that mandates PREA compliance. Because PREA is a federal rule and jails don't receive much federal funding, there is little that the DOJ can do to force compliance. In November 2016, the NYC Board of Correction finally passed the rule making the provisions of PREA local law, albeit with a generous window of time for implementation.[17] Overall, this will be a significant improvement for patients in the city jails, because DOC will be forced to standardize their training, reporting, response, and investigation efforts. But there are still areas of confusion about how this law will be implemented, including the issue of specialized housing areas for transgender patients. When we implemented a voluntary transgender housing area on Rikers, it quickly became a popular and successful unit. In 2012 we embarked on a review of all policies and practices relating to our care of transgender patients, and surveys of patients and staff alike led to the development of the transgender housing area and a complete overhaul of our care to improve access and quality of care for this vulnerable cohort of patients.[18] As of the writing of this book, there is continued discussion at DOC about whether PREA rules either prohibit or support the existence of this critical housing area.

Whether PREA can be interpreted to allow for a transgender housing area or not, the past several years have finally brought the pervasive and unresolved issue of sexual assault in jail into the public eye in NYC. These reform efforts are tremendously important and long overdue, but they will face the uncomfortable truths that every reform can eventually be ignored after a few months or years and that the opinions of security leadership will always outweigh those of the incarcerated. But PREA is a tool we've not had before, a federal mandate (and now local law) on how sexual abuse *must* be addressed and reduced. This is the strongest effort in US corrections to date to mitigate a health risk of incarceration, and it points the way for a broader application of the same idea. People who have their jaw broken or who suffer medical consequences of missed medications or denial of care should be protected in the same manner as those who are sexually abused, and institutions should be required to provide these basic protections as a condition of operation.

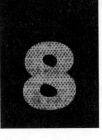

Correctional Health

THERE IS A TENSION in jail health services, because of the ways we are bound to the risks experienced by the incarcerated. In some instances, we're the ones who care for patients after these risks lead to harm. In other circumstances, we're actually part of the risk that incarceration brings. When someone is sent to solitary, or when dual loyalty pressures make us complicit with abuse, we can be part of directly harming our own patients. We've already seen that patients in jail often don't receive the health care they deserve. Now I'll look back at some of the stories we've already examined to focus on how correctional health services in jails can be restructured to reduce health risks to our patients. Because most correctional health services are designed to cut costs and reduce perceived litigation risks, transparency and quality of care are not top priorities. Transforming correctional health is required to reduce the health risks of incarceration, but it is also critical to mitigating our American experience with mass incarceration.

Before diving into the shortcomings of correctional health in this nation, it is important to lay out how correctional health can make a positive difference in the lives of patients. The jail health systems with the best quality and most resources have traditionally been the few that were part of a local public health or hospital system. In these settings, health administrators could make the case that the jail health system was part of the larger community and provide care that addressed chronic medical and behavioral health issues, not just emergencies. With this larger sense of mission, it makes sense to screen and treat for HIV, sexually transmitted diseases like chlamydia and gonorrhea, and also hepatitis C. In our system in New York City, this approach has allowed us to be one of the largest screening/treatment points for asymptomatic men with chlamydia. About 6 out of 100 people screened for chlamydia during jail intake test positive. This sexually transmitted infection often exists without any symptoms in men and is easily treatable with antibiotics. Unfortunately, when left untreated, it can be transmitted to sexual partners rather easily and can cause life-threatening problems such as pelvic inflammatory disease for women and serious eye and lung infections for their newborns. Because unprotected sex is especially common right after leaving jail, we have always been committed to this type of screening and treatment of health problems that other jails avoid based on costs. This approach doesn't reduce mortality in jail and is expensive, but it is critical to protecting partners from infection after jail and reducing the rates of high-risk pregnancy in NYC. This approach to correctional health is often called the public health model and leverages incarceration as an opportunity to improve the health of the incarcerated, as well as that of their families and neighbors. When Dr. Ram Raju was commissioner of health in Chicago, he dramatically expanded Medicaid coverage in Chicago by finding and enrolling people in jail without coverage. Later, as president of NYC Health and Hospitals, he helped us strike a landmark deal with the pharmaceutical company Merck to expand hepatitis C treatment in jail. For the past few years, incredibly effective but expensive medications have been on the market that can cure hepatitis C, which is very common among the incarcerated. Hepatitis C is highly prevalent among intravenous drug users, and as the United States has criminalized drug use, we have driven this cohort of people away from public health settings and toward jails and prisons. This treatment is cost-effective and will reduce the national scourge of cirrhosis and liver cancer, but virtually every jail and most state prisons are resisting this life-saving treatment because of the expense. Taking advantage of the public health opportunities to identify and treat illness among the incarcerated can bring great benefits but is often overlooked because of cost. Unfortunately, this public health approach to jail health care also has a pretty clear limit. It seeks to deliver care to those who often don't receive it, but it doesn't contemplate the harm that jail brings to these same people. In fact, the core assumption in this approach is that we might as well do something worthwhile with people while they're locked up, "turning a negative into a positive," as so many have said. The truth is that these are valuable efforts, but they don't erase the harms of incarceration. And participating in ethical care on one front doesn't excuse ignoring patients on another.

The preceding chapters give a good sense of the ways in which correctional health systems are pressured and manipulated to keep critical information from making its way to outside parties. The most benign view is that correctional health services are innocent but mute bystanders to the health risks of jail. The beating death of young Christopher Robinson in 2008 was the type of case where correctional health might be considered a bystander. His death involved correctional officers who conspired with a group of inmates to open their cell doors and that of Christopher Robinson so they could administer a beating in his cell. This death was ruled a homicide and resulted in criminal prosecutions. For the doctors and nurses in that violent adolescent jail, they reacted to the medical emergency that presented itself and spoke with investigators afterward. Responding to trauma from violence was pretty routine at this time in the adolescent jail. Dr. Tom Freiden, then commissioner of health, pushed us to develop an injury surveillance system that would track and elevate these outcomes to a more senior level. He wanted us to know when our doctors were seeing more patients with broken bones and lacerations so that the leadership in the health service could report back to him and to other leaders in the city about these trends.

We built that proactive surveillance system over the course of five years, and slowly, with the help of the US Department of Justice investigation, the entire city government came to see the value (or necessity) of this aggregate reporting of adverse outcomes. This type of reporting necessarily relies on the health service staff, who know when injuries occur and when those injuries are serious. The same goes for missed medications, self-harm, or sexual assaults. All of this information exists in virtually every jail setting and could be aggregated into rates of outcome for every jail in the nation to report, allowing a real apples-to-apples benchmarking of facility performance. An electronic medical record makes it easier, but either way, it's an embarrassment that we don't have a standardized, transparent, and mandated approach to these health outcomes. We know more about risks from ATV accidents than we do about critical health outcomes that occur during 12 million incarcerations every year in the United States. Creating this type of reporting doesn't eliminate the possibility that security staff might keep patients away from care altogether. In fact, many of the cases in this book reflect this problem. But the lack of transparency in jails about health outcomes is much more consistently tied to losing track of information than actively hiding it. This bureaucratic ineptitude isn't an accident; it's just as intentional as an officer telling a patient to "hold it down" and not go to sick call for a broken nose. But the scale is larger, and it reflects how we have designed jails to operate.

WE'VE SEEN HOW THE Department of Correction can subvert the health service and how individual correctional officers can use caps in the system to hide abuse. But there's another factor that stands in the way of truly reforming the system. Most of the 3,000 jails in the United States deliver health care through contracts with for-profit vendors. This model exists because we've left the funding and oversight of this care to local cities and counties. Thus, the groups that decide how much money to spend, what services should be provided, and how to promote quality are sheriffs and commissioners of correction. There are national jail health standards from groups such as the National Commission of Correctional Health Care, and even guidelines from professional organizations such as the American Public Health Association and the American Medical Association, but these are all voluntary. They are not linked to reimbursement, and there is no consequence to the decision maker for ignoring them. Unfortunately, we've come to accept as a society that community health systems should be mandated to follow evidence-based protocols and reporting, but once patients move into a jail, we are content with unenforceable recommendations that leave health care at the whim of sheriffs and corrections commissioners. The paramilitary organizations that run the jails are focused on security, and their view of health care is extremely narrow and usually limited to preventing death and defending against lawsuits. There are good reasons for security authorities to concentrate on security, but there needs to be someone whose primary concern is to ensure proper delivery of high-quality health care. In Nassau County, New York, the jail moved from having services provided by the local public hospital to a for-profit vendor. One goal of this transition was to reduce hospital transfers and try to manage sick patients more often in the jail. As one might predict, this worked extremely well as a cost-cutting measure and very poorly as a model of care. Several years into this transition, the rate of deaths started to rise, but the sheriff stood by the model, pointing to the millions of dollars saved. By the time this contract was terminated, the rate of death in this jail was several times higher than the national average and the rate in the rest of the NYC jail system.[1]

Breaking the cycle of low-cost and low-quality care in jails is tough, but there are several ways to pursue this goal. The most tried-and-true model is for oversight groups to investigate and mandate improvements, combined with ongoing monitoring by experts. Most jails have experience with this, and the effectiveness of legal sanction and monitoring can range from mild and fleeting to substantial and lasting. In my work in NYC, we have been under settlement agreements ranging from discharge planning for mentally ill patients to access to air conditioning for sick patients to reporting of abuse. These settlements stem from class action lawsuits or investigations by state or federal investigators. Although brutality is a common reason for these suits and settlements, other areas include mandating air conditioning in jails that experience high heat, delivering reentry services to patients with serious mental illness, improving visitation, and improving bathroom facilities. A good friend of mine, Dr. Susi Vassalo, is an emergency medicine physician at NYU/Bellevue and also an expert in a long-standing lawsuit against NYC regarding the lack of air conditioning throughout many of the jails, including most of the solitary confinement areas. This case is similar to many in corrections in that it has dragged on for over a decade and has seen many bureaucratic twists and turns. Part of one phase of agreement was that officers might put trays of ice in front of fans pointed generally toward the cells of inmates instead of NYC simply investing in air conditioning. Eventually, the decrease in solitary use allowed for most people to be transferred to air-conditioned housing areas. I've been inside the solitary cells that lacked air conditioning on warm days, and even for healthy people who may not face risk of heat-related illness, the experience is stifling and maddening. In previous chapters, I have detailed the very welcome investigation by Legal Aid and the DOJ into brutality against our patients. One of the newer examples of this approach is occurring in New York, where the attorney general's health unit has taken individual reports about deaths written by the State Commission on Correction and aggregated systemic concerns about medical care to take actions against substandard correctional health providers. When the attorney general's health unit dives into the health care provided, they often find problems with staffing, quality control, and basic functions like provision of medications. The remedies they have imposed range from traditional monitoring, to fines, to even excluding a vendor from continuing to provide services, as was the case in Nassau County. Unfortunately, none of these measures create a new model of care that isn't profit driven and where the sheriff or DOC is no longer in control of the scope of services and the approach to transparency and quality.

The hope of this strategy is that it pressures the for-profit companies and the various county leaders into providing a more competent level of care. But it has a major weak point. In community hospitals, clinics, and even pharmacies that administer flu shots, there are accrediting bodies that monitor care based on evidence-based measurements, like the Joint Commission, the Center for Medicare and Medicaid Services, and state departments of health. One of the central weaknesses of the oversight that we get, however, is the perpetual reliance on nonmedical entities to improve medical care. Leaving oversight to purely nonmedical entities ensures that only the most egregious failures will be identified, often after systems have declined for years. The difference in approach can be highlighted if we consider the cases of Bradley Ballard and Angel Ramirez, who both died because they became ill and the jail system responded with punishment instead of treatment. In the rest of US medical settings, these types of failures would result in dramatic financial penalties and possible prohibition from further provision of some types of care. In jails, complex patients with alcohol withdrawal, serious mental illness, advanced cirrhosis, or active seizures are routinely held in units that would never pass muster in the community. Somehow, we need to use our success with transparency to advocate for national standards where performance is public and consequences are clear. If every county jail were forced to seek a certificate of approval to house these types of complex patients, or pay for hospitalization, I am quite sure that correctional health competence would increase very quickly—as would diversion of some patients into more suitable settings.

A second, more costly way to improve correctional health is to transfer the health service to a local health department or hospital. This option is usually limited to fairly large cities like New York, Chicago, Dallas, and

Seattle. It can bring more resources and a true sense of quality assurance and improvement, but it's quite a bit more expensive. The single biggest part of this cost is transferring staff from a private vendor with few benefits and no union representation to full civil service titles and benefits. Also, these hospitals rarely want anything to do with correctional health, and once involved, they may turn around and subcontract actual services to the same for-profit vendors they initially replaced. That doesn't seem likely to pass the sniff test, but it is exactly what happened with correctional health the last time it was put into the NYC public hospital system. This model of oversight by a city health agency and care by a for-profit vendor continued when the responsibility went to the NYC Department of Health, but since we've returned to the public hospital system, we have been able to jettison the for-profit vendor and create an entire unified division, much like a new public hospital. This hospital model generally improves the ability to recruit staff and focus on quality assurance and improvement. But the absence of correctional perspective in these institutions can make it difficult to raise issues like dual loyalty, solitary confinement, and brutality. The lack of appetite to discuss critical issues of correctional health can be amplified in public hospitals, where decreasing funding has left most of these institutions on the verge of financial ruin, dependent on local handouts to survive. My central concern for the future of the NYC Correctional Health System is that it will experience a slow erosion of the human rights perspective that was so critical to being an effective advocate for our patients.

Another way to bring in higher-quality care is to create nonprofit correctional health organizations that specialize in this work, like the current for-profits do, but are mission driven and can seek external funding and other benefits of nonprofit health organizations. This model hasn't really taken hold in the United States, but it holds great promise. A great organization in Delaware, Connections CSP, has taken a high-quality community health and social service nonprofit organization and started to provide health services behind bars. In Washington, DC, a collection of local health clinics have come together to provide health services in the district jail. The difficulty with scaling up this nonprofit model is that every local county jail picks their next health vendor based primarily on cost. Still, I believe that this model can work, and it will get a real boost if/when we can crack open the door to Medicaid reimbursement for care inside jail.

An important goal is to connect the funding and quality oversight of jail health care to the rest of the nation. With the opportunity for Medicaid reimbursement, jails could expand their scope of services without new financial investment. Most of the nation's 5,000 jails and prisons have some aspect of health services that they think is important but don't implement, purely because of costs. The availability of outside funding would spur many of them to expand their scope of services as advocates and policy makers apply pressure. But it's the quality oversight that comes with this funding that is the real upside for patients. This idea was proposed to Medicaid officials in 2016, and we were hopeful for results, but the election of President Trump appears to have stalled this effort. Another example of backtracking by the Trump administration relates to the use of private, for-profit prisons. In 2016, President Obama announced a federal ban on for-profit prisons in the federal prison system. Unfortunately, this ban was quickly undone by President Trump, and his comments on criminal justice and immigration foreshadow a return to expanding the number of incarcerated people and utilizing the cheapest means possible to achieve this aim. These recent setbacks paint a bleak picture for the national landscape, but many states have recognized the folly and costs of mass incarceration and are moving to develop drug and mental health courts as pathways toward treatment rather than incarceration. These improvements bode well for correctional health services, since they generally fail to provide anything close to community standards of care for these issues. A more fundamental step, however, would be for states and counties to demand that nonprofit correctional health providers be included in all correctional health contracts. Pressure from the agencies that solicit and pay for these services is needed before community health providers will willingly wade into these troubled waters.

Whatever the model, one feature of community health systems that we can incorporate immediately into correctional health is feedback from our patients. Virtually every clinic and hospital in the United States uses patient surveys about the quality and timeliness of care to guide their operations. These tools were originally called satisfaction surveys but more recently have been thought of as patient experience surveys. Patient experience surveys ask questions about whether health staff listened to patients or explained things clearly to them. In 2015, we conducted the nation's first patient experience survey in a jail, getting the opinions of about 3,000 patients on paper forms. The results confirmed some fears and showed us new areas to concentrate on. For example, when asked about being treated with respect, listened to, or communicated with clearly, about 60 percent of patients fell into the "usually" or "always" categories, with only 10 percent in the "never" groups. But when it came to us keeping health information confidential, the "never" category grew to 20 percent, and only half of respondents felt like we usually or always did so. Also, more than half of patients we surveyed said that they kept health problems from us because they didn't think we would keep them confidential, and more than half also said that they think we (health staff) discuss their health problems with security staff without their permission. Almost one-third of respondents reported not getting the access to sick call that they are guaranteed. In this same survey, we asked about community health engagement and found that over one-quarter of respondents said that time in solitary in jail made them trust doctors outside jail less. This information has helped us to focus on increasing the clarity about what staff can and can't share with security staff, as well renewing our insistence that the security staff should not have access to our EMR, something they often lobby for. The questions we used were standard ones, taken from community surveys used by hospitals and clinics; they could easily be applied to every American jail health service.

There's a third aspect to improving correctional health: the staff. Working in correctional health can be rewarding work, but most correctional health staff toil without the support and training that they need to provide adequate care. Doctors, nurses, and other health staff in jail are very familiar with the brutality, arbitrariness, and unfairness of jail conditions. In most jails and prisons, there is pressure to get along with security staff and little or no effort expended to talk with staff about the real challenges that they and their patients face in promoting health. Like any other profession, when management neglects to acknowledge the real experiences of the staff, they quickly become embittered and start to develop their own approach to their jobs, with a focus on survival and safety. In correctional health, this problem is exacerbated when difficult patients or security staff create a toxic setting that health staff can't address. I recently heard from a physician who had just started working in one of the NYC jails that almost every day correctional officers referred to patients using the "N" word. We've developed forums to discuss these problems in NYC, and while they may not resolve the issues, at least our health staff and their leadership are on the same page about the realities of the work. Around the nation, correctional health staff routinely observe beatings and other physical and verbal abuse of patients. Their reluctance to report these incidents may stem from worry about their own safety, but it also results from years of working in a setting where they soak up the security perspective on their patients and don't get any other message from their leadership.

Journalist Eyal Press published an article in the *New Yorker* in 2015 that focused on abuse of mentally ill patients in the Florida prison system. He homed in on the silence and complicity of health staff, one of whom witnessed a terrible beating of a handcuffed patient by numerous guards. The mental health staffer reported that the lookout of this assault spotted her, and "in the days that followed, the guards involved in the beating dropped by [her] office to tell her that they had 'taken care' of everything. Their tone was polite, but the message was clear, she said: 'We're running this place, this is *our* house—you're just visiting.'"[2] This staffer was warned by colleagues not to report anything, and ultimately, she quit the job. Imagine the staff who stay in these jobs for years. To last, they don't report anything, and any discomfort they feel is bottled up. Acknowledging these problems is difficult when the health authority is independent from the security service, reporting to a separate authority, but it's basically impossible in a for-profit staffing company that earned their contract by being the cheapest bid. It may be that correctional health staff should work in both the community and the jails. That is the way it works in the United Kingdom and several other nations, where there's much less distinction between care inside and on the outside of jails.

In Washington, DC, city officials went through their normal contracting process and selected a for-profit jail health vendor, only to have the city council take the unprecedented step of rejecting the contract. This left the provision of health services in limbo because there wasn't an acceptable alternative. An independent nonprofit could compete with the for-profit vendors and show that better health outcomes are also in the interest of county and security leadership. But creating a new approach to correctional health can do more than reduce the health risks of incarceration; it can also help reduce incarceration. This could be a great time for recruitment to mission-driven correctional health programs, in light of the growing interest in social justice and mass incarceration in the United States. Our correctional health service has been fortunate to recruit newly trained residents and fellows from some of the nation's top programs, including Mount Sinai, Montefiore, and NYU in NYC and the University of California, San Francisco.

Once the independence of correctional health services is assured, then a more community-facing scope of services can be developed. In NYC, we've moved from only providing basic health services inside jail to also doing the brief health screen in Manhattan central booking, which happens hours before decisions about bail or going to jail occur. Pushing into this space with our EMR allows us to do a better job of triaging the people who end up going to jail. But the real benefit for the city is that it allows us to provide some critical information to the patient and their defense lawyer that can lead to treatment for mental health or addiction rather than going to Rikers. Many of our patients have their most reliable health records in the jail EMR, and with their informed consent, we can share that with other social service agencies. On the inside, we have sought and received federal funding to build a large discharge planning service that doubles as a diversion program. The staff who arrange the health services, housing, Medicaid, or food stamps for our patients leaving jail are invaluable assets in helping them avoid jail altogether in the future. Most people in American jails are there because they can't pay for bail and because of the nation's criminalization of drug use and mental illness; most of them cycle in and out of jail as these problems lead them into minor misdemeanor charges and perpetual lack of treatment. Both pre-arraignment screening and in-jail discharge planning programs serve essential functions for people who go to jail, by identifying risk factors for decompensation in the early hours of incarceration and ensuring continuity of care after release. But these programs also represent a key to decarceration. With the involvement of the correctional health program, diversion or alternative-to-incarceration programs can quickly come up with an alternative to bail/jail that involves meaningful treatment.

EVEN IF WE SUCCEED IN REDUCING the nation's appetite for incarceration, we will still have millions of people cycling through jails and prisons every year. It's likely that these people will continue to suffer from high rates of physical and mental health problems, as well as addiction. Creating an independent health authority in each of these places will go a long way toward promoting transparency and ensuring that the health services we design on paper are actually delivered. With 5,000 jails and prisons, there are many types of correctional health systems, but one basic element should exist in every one of them: the health authority should be fully independent of the security service, and security leaders should no more evaluate health care quality or scope of services than they should direct the care of an individual patient.

In the middle of all these issues rests correctional health, a vulnerable and largely compromised institution that is more likely to serve security authorities than patients. While the power dynamic between correctional staff and the incarcerated is understood, the weak position of correctional health is critical to the health risks of incarceration. One tangible example of this imbalance is the medical treatment of correctional officers. Like all correctional health services, we provide emergency treatment to officers in addition to the total spectrum of care provided to the incarcerated. When there is a use of force, however, we are often forced to see less injured officers before more seriously injured incarcerated patients. The way this plays out is that a group of 5–10 officers will come into the jail clinic and take over a cubicle or two and tell the doctor or physician assistant that their colleague needs to be seen. Any patients currently in the clinic will be removed from other cubicles and placed in a pen somewhere. Patients who were injured in the same use of force will not be brought to the clinic until the officers have been treated, and they usually remain hidden away in the intake pens or other places so that our staff often aren't even aware of them until the DOC staff have been cared for. A common scenario will involve DOC staff with hand injuries or muscle strain being seen and treated before an incarcerated patient with facial trauma. The bullying of our staff is so common that when we raise this issue at the highest levels in the city, everyone simply shrugs their shoulders. We haven't had any deaths related to this practice that I'm aware of, but many patients have had to wait for critical emergency care while our staff were attending to lightly injured security staff. In some jails, we try to do both jobs simultaneously, but few jail clinics have this capacity because the security staff usually demand that no inmates be present in the clinic when they are being seen. After a particularly bad episode involving adolescents with head trauma who waited hours for care, I asked our staff to go look for injured patients in the jail intakes whenever they found themselves treating officers in the clinic. We've found many more seriously injured patients this way, but we still rely on DOC cooperation to bring them to the clinic and also to allow emergency medical services into and out of the building, which is another point of intentional and unintentional delay. To be clear, there have been plenty of serious injuries to officers, and we want to treat them first when their injuries merit it. But in jail, almost every injury to an officer is treated before any injury to an incarcerated patient. An additionally subversive aspect of this dynamic is that in NYC DOC staff receive a cash insurance payment any time they go out on an ambulance from work, so our staff were routinely pressured to send officers out for very minor ailments. When our staff have balked, they receive swift retaliation from security staff and even their union leadership. One physician who made the clinical decision that an officer didn't need to go out to the hospital received a profane and intimidating visit to his cubicle by the president of the Correctional Officers' Benevolent Association, Norman Seabrook. Few staff of any type would stick to their clinical judgment with such intimidation, but this provider did. More ominous, though, are the threats to physical safety that can and do ensue when our staff run afoul of the wishes of security staff in these situations. While this is only one example of the power imbalance in jail, it is crucial to understanding how jails harm the incarcerated and then compound those initial harms with barriers to accessing health services.

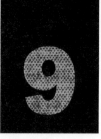

Transparency
and Governance

AMERICAN JAILS ARE horribly run institutions. By design and by incompetence, jails create the risk of death, injury, and illness for the incarcerated. In some jails, like those in New York City, there are so many stakeholders involved that even with more resources, outcomes often appear the same as or worse than we see in other places. In other jails, it's clear that nobody outside the sheriff or Department of Correction has much interest or authority to improve conditions for the incarcerated. The lack of transparency results in reporting by the press that derives from individual bad outcomes or scandals but can't see how pervasive the problems are. In NYC, the jail operations are directed by DOC, while the public hospital system is responsible for health services, but there are many other groups with their hands on the wheel, including unions, oversight bodies, the city council, federal investigators, advocates, legal aid organizations, and an active press corps. With so many agendas in the slow-rolling disaster of the NYC jail system, it has been an agonizing process to reduce the health risks of incarceration to our patients. But we have made substantial gains. Looking back, I believe that our ability to achieve any meaningful improvements has been linked to one principle more than any other: transparency.

Health risks for the incarcerated are directly linked to how secretive a jail is. The sexual abuses of Maria and Brianna share features with the deaths of Christopher Robinson and Bradley Ballard and the assault of Jamal Lightfoot. In each of these cases, security staff were able to have patients moved or isolated in a way that facilitated abuse. Imagine the basic controls that exist in hospitals, hotels, or airports: individual staff cannot take it on themselves to move someone around without supervisors knowing in real-time, or without a record being established. The comings and goings of every housing area in the NYC jail system are monitored via paper logbooks. As you can imagine, the logs are notorious for lacking even the most basic information. There is no clarity about who belongs where at any given time, but the fault is not with the staff who use them inconsistently; the jail leadership have deemed this an acceptable practice. As jail systems like NYC have come under scrutiny for brutality or other problems, rarely have the investigators made information systems a top priority. It's true that the US Department of Justice settlement with NYC did include a significant expansion of cameras, and that is very welcome. But to prevent both abuse and neglect, we could mandate a jail information system that can't be ignored and in so doing create real-time transparency about who is where. For the same reasons, when a health system adopts an electronic medical record, it can be put to use immediately as a potent tool for surveillance of abuse. In NYC jails, DOC's continued reliance on outdated and incomplete paper records and our own aggressive use of the EMR as a human rights tool led to a very lopsided approach to transparency, with the result that the health service is often in the position of knowing and reporting back to the security service how consistently its policies and procedures are being implemented.

Addressing the secretive nature of jails is critical, but so is shining a light on decision-making in oversight bodies. One of the useful features of the NYC Board of Correction is that jail managers must publicly announce or defend their actions to board members, advocates, and the general public. Unlike city council or other infrequent testimony, these meetings occur monthly, and the board members have enough knowledge and data to track progress of reforms and hold us accountable when we fail to meet our goals. In most counties, there is no Board of Correction and no set of rules about custodial or health practices. In NYC, the Board of Correction has rules about security and health practices, and these rules carry the force of law. In March 2012, during my public report to the Board of Correction, I warned that the Mental Health Assessment Unit for Infracted Inmates, a solitary confinement unit for people with mental illness, was an abject failure because of the violence and lack of access to our patients.[1] It would take another year of work, with some tragic outcomes, but with the help of the Board of Correction we closed the unit and designed two alternative approaches.[2] One of the alternatives, designed for patients with less serious mental illness, ended up as a distinction from solitary without a difference, and the Board of Correction would bring in two well-respected experts, Bandy Lee and Jim Gilligan, to catalog the continued practice of punishing patients who required treatment.[3]

The Board of Correction has also been instrumental in keeping the security staff in line with basic standards. Late one Friday in 2014, DOC Commissioner Joe Ponte ordered his staff to transfer mentally ill inmates out of mental health settings and into solitary confinement units if they had unresolved "tickets" for previously breaking jail rules. The second I heard about this, my staff and I told DOC that this would violate city law and their own policies and cause immediate harm and safety risk to patients, officers, and health staff alike. We immediately objected because many of these patients were seriously mentally ill and being cared for in clinical housing areas, but our objections were ignored. The horrible toll this late-night transfer took on patients and staff alike was evident the next morning, when patients who had been stable in treatment settings were floridly decompensating in the chaos of being tossed into solitary units, with no access to medication. When it became clear to even DOC that this move had created massive security and health problems, we spent the following days undoing this blunder. As soon as this incident started to unfold, the Board of Correction communicated to DOC Commissioner Ponte that he was in violation of their rules. This message was repeated a few weeks later when Board of Correction members publicly admonished him for this violation of policy. The discomfort of public humiliation is a strong motivator for security leaders, as well as their bosses in city government. More recently, the Board of Correction has taken the city to task for the long-standing inability to get patients produced for their medical and mental health appointments. The Board of Correction created a public report on access to health services, and being required to own up to these basic failures in public every month has helped us to engage with DOC about the root causes of this problem. Many a time I stood in front of the Board of Corrections being taken to task for a failure of the correctional health service, but never once did I wish the Board of Corrections would become weaker or abolished. Nor did I want them to take on the role of running the health (or security) service. Their strength was as an objective oversight body making the security and health services adhere to minimum standards.

A more traditional approach to improving transparency has been through the many lawsuits and settlement agreements in jails across the nation. Lawsuits often uncover problems, or hints of problems, that lead to official investigations or ongoing monitoring of specific practices. NYC's most recent settlement with the DOJ has brought in a well-respected monitor to head oversight, Steve Martin. Martin started as a correctional officer in Texas and worked his way up the chain of command in corrections, before becoming a consultant and now the nation's most respected court monitor of security practices. Although he works with a pleasant and friendly demeanor, his expertise on monitoring use of force has revealed the ongoing failure of NYC to reform security practices on Rikers. In late 2017, his monitoring team reported that "officers continue to be too rough with inmates who refuse orders or make threats" and that "there's an ingrained propensity of staff to immediately default to force to manage any level of inmate threat or resistance." The core cultural acceptance of violence also appears to remain, with the monitor reporting an "absence of timely accountability for such misconduct."[4]

THERE IS ONE OTHER major factor in promoting jail transparency: the press. Jails are a nonstop source of violent and salacious scandal, and most local papers report on these incidents at one time or another. Reporters Reuven Blau and Graham Rayman have been covering the Rikers beat for more than a decade at the *New York Daily News* and *Village Voice*. In 2008, they wrote a great series on the death of Christopher Robinson. A critical piece by Graham Rayman identified a hidden squad of DOC enforcers that would move in and out of jails without record, administering beatings and "interrogations."[5] Many of the members of this squad would later be indicted and imprisoned for the beating of Jamal Lightfoot. After 2012, a couple of years passed with only sporadic stories about assaults or other incidents appearing in the tabloids, but not much in the way of investigative reporting. One of the troubling aspects of these salacious articles was that they often included photos of injured patients, which were leaked by security staff with incorrect or bigoted perspectives on the patients as the source of the violence. With some security staff eager to leak information that supported their perspective that violence stemmed from the incarcerated, and with no investigation to uncover data that suggested the contrary, DOC practically wrote these stories themselves. This tabloid reporting continues today. A recent article mocked DOC for trying to do something good, with the headline "Rikers Guards to Get Lessons on How to Talk Nicely to Inmates."[6] In fact, DOC was planning to train correctional officers on motivational interviewing, a technique that has been proven to help change behaviors in many settings, even during brief interactions.

The current era of investigative reporting on NYC jails, as well as much of the improved knowledge and awareness of the health risks in these settings, can be attributed to three journalists. First on this modern Rikers beat was Jake Pearson of the Associated Press. When Pearson reported the horrible death of Bradley Ballard, his story was picked up around the nation and quickly crystallized the failures of criminal justice and mental health systems in the United States. Shortly thereafter, he reported on the death of Jerome Murdough, and the attention of lawmakers and advocates was locked on Rikers. As Pearson was starting to cover these and other stories about the jails, the *New York Times* dedicated two investigative journalists to the jail beat, Michael Winerip and Michael Schwirtz. Both journalists knew city politics well, and they slowly dug into the operations of DOC and developed sources there who gave them access to video footage and documents. The first major piece by these two journalists was a two-page spread on brutality. It covered, in part, a detailed report my team and I had written on serious injuries resulting from use of force by correctional officers. We had identified common risk factors for serious injury during use of force and discovered that the patient profiles were of young and mentally ill people, while other variables included being struck in the head or face, being threatened so as not to report injuries or seek care, and being struck after being restrained. We had written the analysis to share with DOC leaders in an effort to reduce injuries, but when it came to light in the *New York Times*, the public was finally able to see how commonplace brutality is in jail. Jumping into jail conditions with both feet, these three journalists continued to develop sources and to report on the systematic risks of incarceration, including shortcomings in our own health service and DOC security practices. Every report by these three journalists made an impression on city government, and much of the support for reform that we have taken advantage of is attributable to them. After Pearson's initial stories broke, a mayoral task force was established to rethink how the city handles criminal justice contact with residents who have behavioral health problems. This task force produced some tangible programs that allowed us to keep people out of jail at best, or improve their care while incarcerated. I've never taken part in another government task force that had such immediate positive results.

Once NYC became focused on the problems at Rikers and the DOJ settlement on brutality was handed down, another crop of journalists came into the picture, focusing on the transition of our health service into the public hospital system and ongoing struggles with DOC. Reporters at *DNAinfo*, *Crain's New York Business*, and local news channels began to regularly cover the jails. Journalists are pulling more of what goes on in jails out into the light and forcing DOC to take an honest look at transparency. But that's not enough, and the press can't do everything.

For every Jake Pearson, Mike Winerip, or Mike Schwirtz, there are dozens of reporters with less time or interest who just need to get a story filed. And for every thoughtful leader or politician like Corey Johnson and Mary Bassett, there are many others who won't bother to dig into the evidence of an issue before making their mind up. Transparency drives reform, but efforts at transparency bring a blend of critiques both fair and unfair, true and untrue. This is one of the tougher parts of governing: keeping focus on a mission while taking incoming fire. When I see the failures around me in city government, it's clear that without the mission to chart our course by, each salvo of criticism can cause a reactive change of course that creates more problems or wastes resources. That kind of reactive policy making drives more decisions than most would suspect, and it's also the reason many talented people leave government. The reason that transparency can't be voluntary is that it often stings and occasionally brings unfair or untrue criticism. I can think of plenty of newspaper articles that reported outright errors or painted a picture that was unfair to our staff, a patient, or someone else. I can't count how many articles have quoted officials from the Correctional Officers' Benevolent Association blaming the health service for violence in the jails, claiming that violence is a product of mental illness and that we in correctional health are either incompetent or unwilling to do our jobs. And there have been times when I stood at the Board of Correction taking public criticism for something that I had no control over. Around the same time that we called out the MHAUII as a failure, we also reported that patients were being moved between mental health units without our agreement or knowledge. Together with my mental health director, Dr. Danny Selling, I had gone to the mat many times on this issue, to no avail. A dear friend and board member, Dr. Bobby Cohen, raised this at a Board of Corrections meeting and admonished us for losing control of our service. The criticism was well deserved, but the power dynamic in the jails was such that if DOC wanted to move someone, there wasn't much we could do to stop it. We felt the sting of that critique deeply, as we did the many others, but the benefit to our patients of more transparency is real and ongoing. There have been many fair critiques of me and our health service. I struggled mightily to explain to Corey Johnson and others in the New York City Council how our use of a for-profit vendor to staff the health service could ever work. In my role working to improve the level of care, we kept adding more quality assurance and clinical oversight of the for-profit company, Corizon, but Councilman Johnson repeatedly circled back to the problem with our basic model: mission-driven oversight of a profit-driven staffing company.

Between 2011 and 2014, we assembled a great deal of data and made proposals on violence and solitary confinement in the jail system, but city hall had scant interest until US Attorney Preet Bharara started his investigation. While good journalism is important and mission-driven oversight is vital, neither is enough to ensure transparency.

There is one vital and missing voice in promoting good governance and transparency: the incarcerated. It's true that advocacy groups like Jails Action Coalition make a strong showing at the Board of Correction meetings, and people with the lived experience also come on their own to comment, but these are viewed by the city and DOC as external voices of dissent, not part of the management apparatus. One of the more chilling exchanges I had in my early years was responding to a suggestion that DOC become part of the Department of Health's Institutional Review Board (IRB). IRBs exist to protect human subjects during research, and ours already comprised formerly incarcerated persons and medical experts with correctional expertise. This suggestion occurred in response to DOC objections to our injury report being published, and my impression was that this was an attempt (unsuccessful) to use the IRB to tamp down our efforts on the health risks of jail.

Inside the jails, each facility has an inmate council that is supposed to meet every month with the jail warden and advocate for improved communication and conditions with the leaders of DOC. My experience in attending these meetings over the years is that the sporadic attendance by DOC leaders and the lack of meaningful records or publication of outcomes are all part of limiting the role of the detained in their own existence. Several years ago, I met with a group of researchers who work in juvenile justice, and they explained the simple but critical metric of perceived fairness among those detainees. Asking the detained about whether they think they're treated fairly seems so simple as to be naive, but in fact, this can be a powerful tool for monitoring how restraint, discipline, and other custodial policies are applied.[7] Just as injuries and other health consequences of jail must be tracked and reported from every facility, basic information from detainees should be collected and reported. The ideal of transparency would incorporate not only objective health outcomes like preventable deaths and injuries but also the same types of perceptions about care and conditions that every hospital and clinic is obliged to survey, including whether one is treated with respect or whether medical decisions are explained. But these types of innovations aren't likely without legal mandates that make them both uniform and universal. I don't think that transparency is enough to eliminate the health risks of incarceration, but it is absolutely essential to the task. There are strong examples we can rely on, but they require substantially more commitment than we've shown as a nation. When we started to focus on patients injured in uses of force at Rikers, we devised our clinical encounters after the tool we'd learned to use to evaluate survivors of torture, called the Istanbul Protocol.[8] That tool, used by doctors around the world since 1999 to document torture and abuse, also comes with a raft of structures and protocols for how governments and nonstate actors need to oversee security services, jails, and prisons to ensure that torture does not occur. This approach involves setting up something called a "national protective mechanism" that enables groups of experts to visit any detention facility unannounced and monitor for human rights violations. This is akin to the work of the International Committee of the Red Cross, but findings aren't bound to secrecy, and the point of these visits and oversight is to bring problems into public light. Imagine how many of the needless deaths recounted in this book and that occur in other jails would have been prevented if every state had a group of independent doctors and lawyers visiting jails and prisons unannounced and reporting publicly on their findings. The Istanbul Protocol, which we used as a template for our efforts in Rikers, is only one small part of this approach. Setting up and funding all the structures needed for a national plan to end torture is something the US government and states have resisted, even as this approach has been implemented in Europe and elsewhere. The lack of a US commitment to ending torture means that efforts to bring abuse to light like ours only occur sporadically and may not even endure changes in leadership or public interest.

The second critical element to this mission is leadership. In virtually every bad outcome portrayed in this book, there was an opportunity for someone to step in and stop events or redirect them to a better outcome. I have been in the room when commissioners of agencies, wardens of jails, and chief medical directors of hospitals kept quiet while unethical or misguided policies were being promoted. Similarly, in most of the positive outcomes I portray here, someone did take a position that would bring pressure or scorn. When Commissioner Farley gave me the green light to publish the injury data in 2012 and the solitary data in 2014, he knew we would both pay a price for it with city hall and DOC. When his successor, Dr. Mary Bassett, came to the jails to help us correct the placement of seriously mentally ill patients in solitary, she also paid a price with the orchestrated and public dressing-down by Norman Seabrook, the now-indicted correction officers' union boss. The multiple public attacks on her by Seabrook elicited scant defense by a city hall administration that was clearly rankled by her use of science and data to advocate strongly on behalf of the detained.

There were several times when we in the correctional health service raised an alarm that required the response of others, including sharing data concerning sexual assaults, sharing data on the health effects of solitary confinement, and most prominently when we wrote the use-of-force report and shared it widely across DOC. The unwillingness of the city government to deal with these issues opened the door for US Attorney Preet Bharara to become involved. Once the press stories and the DOJ investigation came into the light in 2014, our need to conduct analyses of patient injuries and other forms of abuse in the dark gave way to broader acceptance of our approach of documenting the harms of jail. But beforehand, a relatively small group of us in correctional health worked to find and report cases and trends of abuse, and we partnered with Cathy Potler and Bobby Cohen at the Board of Correction, Jonathan Chassan and others at Legal Aid, and a few others to make sure that abuse was reported and that the groups responsible for investigating abuse were held accountable. A review of the coauthors on the 40 or so papers we published during this time will reveal the key members of our team. That group represents the finest example of health advocacy that I have ever been a part of; for many, their involvement felt like a great professional risk, and their accomplishments in documenting and reducing the health risks of jail have laid a path for others to follow across the nation.

One of the lessons I've learned in leading this team has been the special role that physicians have in promoting social justice. We have a great deal of clout, both earned and unearned, when we voice our opinions. When we use our skills in epidemiology and medicine together with the principles of human rights, we can make a substantial contribution to improving the lives of our patients, especially when we partner with legal and social work groups. When Megan McLemore from Human Rights Watch wrote a report about the NYPD using condom possession as a pretext to arrest women for sex work, I was just as appalled as other New Yorkers. She and other advocates, including Kate Mogulescu from Legal Aid, were working to end this practice, which involved not only using condom possession as a pretext for arrest but also the habit of police stopping and searching women and throwing away or taking their condoms.[9] Not only did this fly in the face of one of the most successful public health interventions in history, but it also seemed to target a group of vulnerable women. When we heard about this, we quickly looked at the rates of sexually transmitted infections among women in jail and saw significantly higher rates among those charged with sex work–related crimes. Although we were late to this fight, our subsequent report added a piece of evidence against this practice from the same city administration that was implementing it.[10] This approach doesn't necessarily change minds, but it does put city lawyers on notice that medical experts are at odds with a city practice. The same approach helped to eliminate the MHAUII because the defense of that practice was undercut by data from the city's own experts in correctional health. For struggles like these, physicians can bring attention that's hard to ignore, even if they aren't first to the fight or even the loudest voice.

ANOTHER ADVANTAGE OF promoting human rights as an American physician is our ability to find another job if we are fired for taking a stand. This isn't so true for other types of staff, and it also isn't true for physicians working in other nations. The worst pushback I've ever received to the work described in this book involved a little physical intimidation, threats to my job, and nasty emails. Mostly, the result of our work has involved gripes to higher-ups about me and our team. But physicians I've worked with from Iraq, Egypt, Turkey, Jordan, Uganda, and other settings face far direr consequences when they stand up for their patients. For them, effective leadership may be less about starting fights with the overwhelming authority of their governments and more about minimizing harm and documenting abuse in a way that keeps them and their patients safe.

In the past year with Physicians for Human Rights, I've been in many spots where torture and sexual violence are ongoing and where doctors risk their lives and those of their families by speaking up. I was recently near Mosul just after the fall of ISIS, and the doctors who emerged from that horror related stories of survival and commitment to their patients that shook everyone within earshot. But because of our job security and social status, physicians in the United States have a doubly privileged position, and we can put it to good use. Most of the time, we can improve the lot of our most vulnerable patients through training our own colleagues and also forging partnerships with social workers, nurses, and others who have a closer view of social inequities and discrimination. There are also times when we need to put our credibility on the line and step into charged conflicts.

When I was a boy, my father would sometimes get threatening phone calls about testifying in child abuse cases. Although his status as a physician gave important credibility to the justice process for abused children, it also made him a public target. Most of the time, however, our special role as physicians will mean steering policy decisions in a direction that helps our staff and patients come together in a more equitable or humane manner. A contemporary example is the wholesale change in our correctional health model in the NYC jails. We had long advocated for a new model to correctional health in NYC that would end the reliance on a for-profit vendor to provide staffing and would instead create a mission-driven nonprofit service. We actually planned this as the next step of improvement in the DOHMH, but city officials would decide that correctional health must be transferred back to the public hospital system. In the transition from our model of DOHMH/Corizon to the public hospital system, it has been inspiring to see how our leaders of the nursing, mental health, and medicine services breathed new life into staff who hadn't previously been very well engaged. These leaders, Nancy Arias, Ross MacDonald, and Elizabeth Ford, have been able to engage with their staff, recruit new mission-driven deputies, and make dramatic improvements to how our health service works. Their commitment to caring for our patients is clear, and they have transformed the service into one where people are proud to work and that newly trained doctors, nurses, and social workers are eager to join. This team is a rarity in correctional health in any nation, but it could be the norm if we can address the many issues facing correctional health. But the challenge will still be to force DOC and city officials to take their mission seriously. Their battles will hopefully be less about brutality and solitary confinement and more about improving the system until it resembles care in the community. The perilous state of the city's public hospital system will make them a ripe target for raiding staff and funds. The DOC will continue to seek control over the health service through an outright takeover or by subversive changes like gaining access to the EMR. These and other struggles will fall to the correctional health team. Their capacity to continue reducing the ways in which the jail system harms patients will rest on their leadership skills and on the level of transparency that can be achieved across the jail system.

Although most people in jail are charged with minor crimes, they contend with serious health risks created by the jail, including death, injury, and sexual assault. Kalief Browder, Bradley Ballard, and the many others profiled in this book suffered because of the systemic harms created in the NYC jail system. Every jail has its own profile of harm, but before we can eliminate or reduce the risks, we need to be honest about what they are. We need to develop more independence in the jail health services, so that care will not be negatively influenced by security priorities and so that reliable data can be collected and reported. Without reliable information, we only learn of the health risks of jails when things go horribly wrong, and without credible transparency, suspicion of wrongdoing or incompetence will be assumed.

The first step toward reducing the health risk of jail is to establish standards in reporting health outcomes. Already, we have some death data sporadically reported through the DOJ. In addition, with jails moving toward PREA compliance, we are starting to see aggregate reports on sexual abuse. These data are available, but not in a format that allows stakeholders like city council or state policy makers to compare one jail to another or track trends over time. Also, we need to report the subset of deaths that are "jail-attributable." This should include all suicides, homicides, and early-admission deaths because the first 72 hours represent a time when death is often the result of failures in the intake process, as was the case for Mr. Mercado. Additionally, we still don't see any data outside NYC on injuries and physical or mental health episodes stemming from missed medications. Aside from these health outcomes, we also need to see concrete numbers on critical processes, such as percentages of appointments that are kept or percentages of medications that are administered on time (see table A.2). In NYC, council members Corey Johnson, Danny Dromm, and their colleagues developed a number of bills to mandate public reporting of these types of outcomes in city jails.[11] This approach could be easily implemented in other settings, with attention to outcomes and methods that can be compared across jails. Although it would be far more efficient and helpful if the Centers for Disease Control or the DOJ were to mandate such an approach, this seems unlikely given the current political climate. Conversely, with many cities and counties expressing frustration with their jail systems, there may be an opportunity to provide technical assistance to local oversight bodies to enact the types of reporting we have in NYC and then rely on academic partnerships to aggregate these data.

As in any human rights endeavor, documenting problems doesn't fix them and may bring retaliation before it brings a willingness to change. In NYC we certainly experienced plenty of pushback and discontent over our early reporting on injuries and solitary confinement. But the more settings that publicly report data, the more likely that rates of health outcomes can be used to show progress, not just document failures. For example, once we can get the largest 25 jails reporting death and injury rates, we will be able to show who is above and below the median, and when a serious injury occurs during a use of force, the well-performing jail will have more to respond with than "the Commissioner cares deeply about every inmate and has zero tolerance for abuse of . . ." Similarly, when we identify jails that perform poorly and do not improve, we should use those data to push the discussion about closing the facility. Hospitals and clinics are not allowed to stay in business if they repeatedly fail their inspections. Because jails are local institutions, many poorly run or poorly designed jails have operated for decades because the local officials have suppressed transparency or thwarted accountability. For state attorneys general and the DOJ, having standardized outcomes data would enable them to push for corrective actions before class action or other legal proceedings ensue.

The benefit of transparency about the health risks of jail will go well beyond jail administration, however. Some of the nation's most powerful entities are health insurance companies and health systems. These organizations have been largely silent on mass incarceration, but they are waking up to the grim economic realities driven by mass incarceration. Patients who go to jail have high rates of substance abuse disorder, mental health problems, and chronic medical problems. One disease, hepatitis C, is providing an unwelcome orientation to the health risks of incarceration for these powerful groups. Hepatitis C is a chronic infection transmitted via blood and body fluids and is very common among people with criminal justice involvement. Hepatitis C infection can seem to have little impact on a person until decades later, when the dreaded complications of liver cancer or cirrhosis may appear. For the first time, we now have medications that can cure hepatitis C; this treatment is very expensive but also highly cost-effective.[12] But because local jails have to pay for care of the incarcerated, there is heavy pressure to avoid treatment based solely on cost. Additionally, for the patients who are initiated on this expensive but effective treatment in the community, they are likely to have their medications interrupted while in jail, potentially requiring a restarting of therapy. This type of cost to community insurers or health systems is critical to document so that we can bring these parties to the table when discussing criminal justice reform. Much of the criminal justice reform in sentencing, and even in solitary confinement, has been driven by states wanting to reduce their staffing costs. In this manner, clearly documenting the health risks of mass incarceration to the parties that pick up the tab will encourage them to rethink our overall approach. The complexity and cost of these units should help us to rethink whether or not we should be jailing seriously mentally ill people, but they shouldn't force us to capitulate to a lesser standard. Our hospitals, blood banks, clinical laboratories, and other health settings all operate on the requirement that they have a set level of staffing, equipment, and quality control. We should have the same expectation of our jails, and failures to meet standards should result in jails losing their ability to function. Not only do we need full and appropriate teams, but we also need to give them evidence-based training such as crisis intervention for health and security staff to reduce the use of force. Health staff need standardized dual loyalty training and support to help them report abuse and neglect. I am quite confident that in almost every one of our 5,000 American jails and prisons health staff turn a blind eye to abuse and neglect because their mission has been overwhelmed by the security service.

Conclusion

What to Do with Rikers

In 2016, discussions about the future of Rikers moved into full public view. The city has considered closing Rikers for more than a decade, but the political and financial cost of moving operations off the island was always a deal breaker. After the tragedies of Kalief Browder, Bradley Ballard, and so many others had worked their way into the mainstream thanks to aggressive investigative reporting, the continued failures of the Department of Correction to reduce violence and the Department of Justice investigation made closing Rikers a prominent question in the public domain. Closing Rikers even became a point of conflict in the ongoing struggle between New York governor Andrew Cuomo and New York City mayor Bill de Blasio, further elevating the issue. My view is that Rikers should be closed. Many of the reasons that the NYC jail system continues to fail at its core missions of care, custody, and control flow from the enormous scale of Rikers, the crumbling physical plant, and the feudal nature of the individual jails. Closing Rikers requires building one or two new jails, but this is required anyway, so the question is whether they should be on Rikers or not. Having spent the past eight-and-a-half years struggling to provide and improve health services in this system, I am convinced that the path to a more humane and less harmful jail system requires closing Rikers.

The question about closing Rikers has become such a hot topic that the two principal policy makers in New York have weighed in on predictably opposite sides of the issue. Part of the DOJ's direction to the city as a result of their brutality findings was to get adolescents off Rikers because the setting was too violent and abusive for them. The cascade of public opinions on closing Rikers started in April 2016, when then city council chairwoman Melissa Mark-Viverito declared closing Rikers as a goal and announced a commission to study the matter. Shortly thereafter, Governor Cuomo declared closing Rikers to be a great idea, followed 24 hours later by the mayor stating that it was unrealistic.[1] This spat was further sustained with highly scrutinized statements in favor of closing Rikers by the mayor's wife, Chirlane McCray, and the NYC comptroller, Scott Stringer.[2] Shortly thereafter, Stringer published a damning report on the NYC jail system that revealed increasing violence despite a record low inmate census and record high spending and numbers of correctional officers. Although the matter is far from settled, the de Blasio administration has signed on to the idea of closing Rikers, and in early 2018 the city announced that one of the jails on Rikers will close in the summer of 2018, as the census fell below 9,000 for the first time in recent history.[3]

The conventional wisdom regarding closing Rikers is that, having gone from over 20,000 people in jail in the 1990s to about 9,000 today, we could reduce this even more to about 6,000. If we get to this point, we could then build another jail or two off Rikers with a total capacity of 2,000–3,000, and we could also use the existing jails in Manhattan, Brooklyn, and the Bronx and maybe reopen the one in Queens. There would be significant expense to building these new facilities and even more to knocking down everything on Rikers and then realizing the benefits of either real estate development or expansion of LaGuardia Airport. This broad plan is achievable, but the barriers are immense. Earlier in 2016, Mike Winerip and Mike Schwirtz at the *New York Times* summed up the issue correctly: "Close Rikers Island? It Will Take Years, Billions and Political Capital."[4] The challenges to closing Rikers are both complex and deep. No local legislator wants a jail in their neighborhood, and the ability of local community boards to block the closure of a failing hospital for years is a recent cautionary tale for anyone looking to drop a jail into an unreceptive neighborhood.[5] NYC officials have worked on multiple options for changing the jail system, including refurbishing the jails on Rikers, partially closing some of the nine jails being used, or completely closing the jails and relying on existing and new off-island facilities. The political ramifications of even discussing a new jail are so sensitive that the mayor's senior staff initially denied that they had taken any concerted effort toward developing alternate plans before a PowerPoint presentation was leaked to the press that involved five city agencies and was titled "Alternatives for Rikers Island." This presentation was politically charged because it identified a site in Brooklyn and another in Staten Island as potential locations for new jails.[6] Since that time, politicians from the neighborhoods in question have weighed in against the plan, so for now the question is an academic one.

But aside from local objections to building new jails and the cost of those facilities, there's an equally tough challenge in reducing the overall jail population. NYC is in somewhat uncharted territory, having already reduced the rates of incarceration more than any other large American city. A large measure of this success has been achieved through changing prosecutorial practices around minor offenses like marijuana possession, as well as development of programs that steer people with mental illness and addiction problems into treatment instead of jail. The diversion to treatment programs has relied on the participation of several key judges in administering drug or mental health courts that can review misdemeanor and even felony cases and work with social and health service organizations to establish treatment. These efforts can be expanded, but they require more consistent practices by prosecutors and judges and, importantly, increased community resources for addiction and mental health treatment. The resource most lacking, but essential to the success of diversion programs, is supportive housing. Dr. Ross MacDonald's analysis of Rikers frequent flyers was featured in the *Wall Street Journal* and revealed a cohort of 800 people who averaged only 31 days between incarcerations, almost always for minor misdemeanors.[7] Two things stood out about this group: high rates of homelessness and addiction. Incarceration isn't serving any purpose for this group, but repeated contact with police for minor nonviolent crimes leads them right back to jail. We've started working with the Manhattan district attorney and other agencies to find supportive housing for these people as a way to reduce their chances of returning to jail, but the space available is far outpaced by the need. Expanding this approach would reduce recidivism and the overall jail population by about 1 in 10. An important method that's helped us get this far has been to leverage our reentry team in the health service as a diversion resource. Many of these patients have most of their medical records in jail, and our staff routinely participate in diversion plans.

Many people go to jail simply because they are poor and can't make bail. Bail is intended to ensure appearance at trial, nothing else. In theory, people who might skip out on their trial should receive high bail and others lower or no bail. In reality, bail is what keeps the poor (mostly people of color) in jail while those with money go home to await trial. Kalief Browder's bail of $3,000 might as well have been $3 million for his mother. The same goes for Jerome Murdough, who died at Rikers after being arrested for sleeping in the stairwell of a public housing complex on a cold winter night and receiving bail of $2,500. In response, the NYC Mayor's Office of Criminal Justice has rolled out a new supervised release program that will keep about 3,000 people out of jail each year, which could decrease the annual admissions to jail by about 6 percent and the daily census from 10,000 to 9,400. The city has also initiated a smaller program to pay bail for some people who cannot afford it.[8] In tandem with these bail initiatives, Mayor de Blasio announced a "justice reboot" in 2015 aimed at shortening the length of time people wait for trial, with special emphasis on 1,400 people like Kalief Browder— defendants waiting in jail for more than a year for resolution of their case.[9] Over the first 18 months, this program did succeed in resolving some old case backlogs, but the pace of newly languishing cases continued, and the number of people waiting a year at Rikers is still about 1,400.[10]

ULTIMATELY, THESE PROGRAMS will nibble at the problem but won't fundamentally reduce the Rikers population. The racial unfairness of bail is well documented, and the objective of bail, to ensure that people show up for trial, can easily be met without incarceration since the overwhelming majority of people released to the street after arrest show up for their court dates.[11] A few cities, such as Washington, DC, have abolished money bail in favor of a set of rules about pretrial detention that are unrelated to the ability to pay.[12] This innovation reduces incarceration and saves money, but it makes judges and prosecutors nervous because they lose the ability to investigate cases while defendants are locked up or to coerce guilty pleas from people desperate to return home from Rikers. Also, there is a political risk to promoting a fairer approach for tens of thousands because of the eventuality that some out awaiting trial will be charged with new crimes. In Washington, DC, this happened about 10 percent of the time. About 40 percent of inmates in the NYC jail system are there because they can't pay bail.[13] If we can eliminate money bail in NYC, this group of about 4,000 represents the real potential for making a significant reduction in the jail population and closing Rikers.

Because the NYC jail system creates health risks for the incarcerated, we should develop new approaches to criminal justice that eliminate or reduce those risks. NYC, like many cities and counties, turned its back on jail conditions for years, and a culture of mismanagement and brutality took hold that has not been removed. The sheer size of the NYC jail system makes it virtually unmanageable, and the way that the jails function as local fiefdoms encourages dumping of patients who are viewed as problematic on other jails. This tendency results in some of the most challenging and highest-need people in the jail system spending large amounts of time in jail intake pens or otherwise being abused or neglected, which is the opposite of what evidence tells us they require: structured management plans, medication adherence, and consistent rules enforcement. If we were able to reduce the overall daily jail census to 5,000 or 6,000, then a small number of jails could operate in a specialized manner, with a clear set of rules about which patients go to which facility. Mark Cranston, a colleague of mine, was the first deputy commissioner at NYC DOC and is now the warden of the Middlesex County Jail in New Jersey. We've often talked about the challenges in running Rikers, and although we have different perspectives on some issues, we always agree on the need to transform the NYC system so that a small number of wardens are empowered to remake the culture in their jails, with the confidence that the DOC leadership won't torpedo their efforts with endless transfers into and out of their facilities.

Assuming that one isn't advocating total abolition of jail, we should enforce minimum requirements for jails to ensure that their tendency to harm the incarcerated is measured, reported, and minimized. The NYC Board of Correction has made great strides in forcing DOC to improve, but they face a city government and DOC that seem content to receive citation after citation for failing to meet minimum standards. The work of the Board of Correction has been greatly assisted by the pressures of the DOJ investigation and PREA legislation. But two critical challenges remain on the back burner: a deteriorating physical plant in most jails, and a backward approach to information management. This inability to provide a safe and constitutional level of custody must be addressed as we also try to further reduce incarceration rates.

Most NYC jail detainees are in housing areas and intake pens that are so decrepit that weapons can easily be fashioned from parts of the wall, ceiling, plumbing, and light fixtures. Staff and other patients are usually around inmates who are armed, and there's almost nothing to be done about it. In addition, even when DOC and health staff agree that a patient requires a higher security setting, DOC may transfer them to an isolation cell or other setting that fails to meet security needs and also makes provision of health services impossible. The lack of secure and humane housing drives many of the conflicts about whether or not patients are receiving mandated services. In addition, many of the jail's housing areas lack fire safety, air conditioning, and other basic requirements. Once, during a fire, the jail was chaotic as security staff moved groups of inmates away from the fire and NYC Fire Department trucks rolled onto the island. I went to each of the housing areas near the fire to make sure nobody was still locked in. Afterward, an FDNY official told me that the modular building was "like a papier-mâché box with 1500-pound air conditioners on top; I won't send my guys in there if it's on fire." There are areas where patients are held in cells with broken windows, inoperable toilets, or other basic deficiencies that reflect custodial failure. The medical infirmary was literally the DOC bus garage before they decided to upgrade their bus fleet to another site and hand the space over to us for our sickest patients. I've often heard complaints about inmates who would file lawsuits about bits of the ceiling material falling down on them, but the scope of the problem became clear to me when we received a report that a rotting animal carcass had fallen into the patient area.

Another physical plant shortcoming throughout the jails is the lack of appropriate single-cell settings. We have a couple of jails with good housing areas where patients can be secure in a cell of their own at night but out and participating in multiple programs in day rooms and open areas during the day. But more often, our single-cell areas are built for solitary confinement, with little congregate or program space. We have so much housing stock without air conditioning that we and DOC engage in a clumsy effort every summer to get the patients with chronic health issues transferred into air-conditioned housing areas. One of the barriers to moving the adolescents off island, as indicated by the DOJ, has been a lack of space for school in the existing jails in Manhattan and Brooklyn, so the near-term plan is to house them in existing juvenile justice facilities under DOC custody pending their total transfer to custody of the Administration for Children's Services.[14] The inadequacies of physical plant and information management warrant closing several current jails and building one or more new jails, including new spaces that can bring programs and engagement to everyone while safely and humanely housing special populations like high-security inmates and infirmary patients. There are some parts of the jails that meet the needs of staff and patients, including the women's jail, which has a good infirmary, nursery, and new housing area building. But the norm for most jails is a decrepit physical plant and unending "projects" to bring the jails up to the bare minimum standards of safety and efficiency.

As I've laid out in prior chapters, the deteriorating facilities are matched by an archaic paper-based approach to information management that may be the single greatest contributor to abuse and neglect in the jails. The NYC jail system has more correctional officers than inmates, and with all of those resources, we still don't know in real time how to find all of our patients. In this book I've presented a number of completely preventable deaths that occurred in the intake corridor of the system's largest jail, the Anna M. Kross Center. Patients arrive on a bus and cycle through a series of pens as they work their way down the corridor after each security step. They are also brought there after incidents out in housing areas, sometimes to be forgotten or further punished. Distressingly, almost nobody could tell you who is in each pen, and when a bus rolls up to disgorge 5 or 25 inmates, there is no list of who is on the bus. Patients have individual ID cards, their names are written on a list by hand, and their progress from pen to pen is hopefully tracked on paper logbooks, as is their progress over to the medical clinic for their intake physical. For the patients who are brought there from housing areas after a use of force, there is supposed to be a logbook record of when they arrive and when they leave, but as we have seen for years, patients often languish for hours in these pens waiting for medical care. We noted this issue in our use-of-force report in 2014, but in those cases we interpreted the delays as part of retaliation. The problems reported by the current DOJ monitor point to a more pervasive issue: the basic inability to track the movement of injured patients from one part of the jail to another and get them access to care. While this particular intake corridor can boast plenty of mismanagement, one of the core issues is the jail itself. I have been to other jails where people move from bench to bench during their intake. With this approach, it's much more apparent when someone is sick or over-dosing, and pens are only used for short periods of time and for patients who pose a safety risk. Also, most jails have a way to track inmates more akin to an emergency room, so that the number of people in the intake and their identities are available at the click of a button. Importantly, this type of system can also let supervisors (and their leadership) see when anyone is in the intake for more than an hour or two, especially if they're waiting for a medical encounter.

Beyond the questions of reducing incarceration and improving conditions of confinement, there's also the issue of the Rikers culture. The DOJ investigation noted this, as has every comprehensive look at brutality and neglect in the NYC jails. There is a deeply ingrained ethos that relies on violence and intimidation to conduct the business of the jails. As the city government refused to acknowledge the problems with brutality and also failed to engage with the correction officers' union on this issue, the culture of violence was baked into the jails. This culture of violence was a primary reason for my team to adopt our human rights framework to correctional health. The widespread acceptance of using violence against patients was a defining feature of the jail system when I took over the health service, and all of the power and organization seemed to lie with the groups promoting this approach, while the critics of brutality seemed weak and ineffective. But there have been important improvements in the culture: many of the leaders and practitioners of the culture of violence are gone, some even incarcerated; reliance on solitary confinement and violence by correctional staff is dramatically decreased; officers are receiving training in crisis intervention; and more cameras are being installed. The officers and leadership of DOC now feel the consequences of using excessive force against our patients.

But engagement of officers is very low, and violence against them and between patients remains high. If you ask officers, they will tell you that the loss of solitary and "enforcement" (a euphemism for "judicious" beatings) has brought chaos and left them unwilling to do their jobs for fear of prosecution. That they feel unsafe and persecuted cannot be ignored. The same problems with basic jail management that create health risks for the incarcerated also impact staff. The officers who work in the AMKC intake corridor have no reliable way to know who is in what pen and who has been there too long. As a result, everyone yells and screams at them, and they deal with constant verbal and physical abuse. In addition, the new tools that will help avoid violence, like crisis intervention teams and our new mental health units, have been rolled out in only a small number of places, leaving most officers with little view of improved conditions and skeptical of what they do see. Recently, in the midst of the DOJ monitoring of use of force, the DOC leadership brought in a consultant to teach use of new weapons, including Tasers and shotguns that could use both lethal and nonlethal ammunition. This consultant was essentially run off Rikers Island by the security staff he was there to train, and the acrimony seemed attributable to this very credible complaint of officers: they're not part of decision-making, and they are the ones who pay the price for managerial incompetence.[15]

The disconnect between managers and line staff has been further exacerbated by the Correctional Officers' Benevolent Association, which is eager to blame violence on mental illness and failures of the health service. In a recent statement, the president of COBA asked, "How then is it that someone with the record of violence can continue to refuse treatment and lash out at will? Why have we not investigated medical solutions to these violent mentally unsound individuals? The violence caused, as well as destruction to city property exhibited, are NOT the actions of individuals NOT suffering from mental health problems. Can we not find mental health solutions such as they do with violent inmates in other jurisdictions?"[16] My initial reaction to this rant was to be angry that our patients and our mental health service were being misrepresented. This is essentially the same line COBA has taken for the past decade, even when horrible uses of force or assaults on their officers clearly didn't involve anyone in the mental health service. Also, our data clearly show that seriously mentally ill patients are involved in fewer uses of force and incidents of violence than in prior years owing to recent improvements. In fact, the growth in jail-based violence has been among those NOT in the mental health service. But I'm reminded that connecting with people's frustration and fear is often more motivating than having an accurate handle on what caused those problems, or what will fix them. This myth about the mentally ill causing surges in violence isn't any closer to the truth than the last 10 times it has been propagated by COBA, but what matters is that the union works to connect with the officers about how they feel: unappreciated, angry, and afraid. They have also worked very effectively in labor negotiations with the city, so COBA now bargains at the same table with the police officers' union. Although I have crossed swords with COBA over their scapegoating of our patients or staff, the concerns of their officers aren't any less real. Somehow, we've managed to implement reforms that address some critical areas of the jails but still don't resolve these sentiments. All of this bears on the issue of the culture of Rikers. If I had to wrap up what the culture really has been over the past decade, it's one of mismanagement. If you strip away the location and the job descriptions and the horrible tragedies, Rikers has suffered from years of weak and ineffective management from multiple mayors on down through their deputies and the corrections commissioners and their senior staff. The leaders of the brutality in 2011–2014 were promoted in the prior years because their approach seemed most effective to the leadership of NYC, as well as that of DOC and COBA. By the time this approach was completely out of control, other real problems like the deteriorating physical plant and lack of information systems had fallen off the table, and there was no alternative management approach ready to implement. This isn't to say that the cultural acceptance of violence doesn't persist. The DOJ monitor has noted in his most recent report a troubling persistence of "head shots" during uses of force. This was a major finding of our use-of-force report in 2014, and even as we roll out new tools like crisis intervention training and better mental health units, the tendency of staff to strike patients in the head hasn't been eliminated.[17]

In late 2016, the NYC comptroller, Scott Stringer, released a harshly critical report on the status of reforms in the jails.[18] While this type of report should be viewed in a political context, with the comptroller a critic and potential challenger to the mayor, the statistics in the report are halting. The number of people in the city jails in 2016 was the lowest in 33 years, yet the number of officers had grown by over 2,000 since 2014, reaching a ratio of more than 1:1 for officers and inmates. The annual cost per inmate increased by 37 percent during this period, reaching $132,019. All of this would be tolerable if these investments achieved the stated goals of safer jails, but as the report documents, "the rate of fight/assault infractions reached 1,148 per 1,000 average daily population in Fiscal Year 2016, representing an increase of 25% over the prior year, 48% over the last two years, and 144% since 2007." In addition, concerns about how accurately these incidents are reported continue to persist with ongoing allegations that these numbers are manipulated.[19]

WE NEED TO CLOSE RIKERS. We have worked for many years to document and reduce the harms that the jail system creates for our patients, but the harmful mix of mismanagement, inadequate physical plant and information system, and isolation of Rikers all remain. Unfortunately, these jails are short on programming space and other modern jail features, so there will be a need for at least 2,000–3,000 beds in new facilities. This likely involves at least two new jails, including a facility for women. The power dynamic between eager real estate developers and reluctant neighborhood advocates is one that I'm not expert in, much like the wrangling between the governor, the current mayor, and their potential challengers. But no matter what, NYC needs new jail facilities, and it certainly makes more sense to locate them off Rikers and to force ourselves to innovate in both our custodial practices and information management. I don't think that simply building a new jail or two and repurposing what we have in the boroughs would address the health risks of jail, but it would make the problems much more manageable.

With nine jails operating on Rikers, there is a constant need for repairs of leaking roofs and burst water mains. Fire safety remediation and unending plumbing and construction problems leave the facilities pitted against each other for resources. Having developed a new, evidence-based approach to mental health care in our PACE units, and having received ample funds for more units, we have found ourselves unable to roll out new units in a timely manner because we and DOC can't find safe housing areas. Even when we do identify an appropriate setting, the DOC construction staff needed to make critical safety modifications to these units are often overwhelmed with other physical plant emergencies and construction obligations of various settlement agreements. At a recent city council hearing, council member Corey Johnson acknowledged the virtue of our new PACE units but homed in on the fact that most patients with serious mental illness are not in these dramatically improved units. I had to acknowledge that

only about 200 of the 900 seriously mentally ill inmates were in these housing areas. Our new funding to expand this model further envisions another
two units per year, but this will take many years. As Councilman (now City
Council Speaker) Johnson reminded me and everyone else, the slowness of
that plan, even with funding, leaves hundreds of vulnerable people in settings we know to be unsafe.

Overall, we have built a number of successful new programs and units,
like Clinical Alternative to Punitive Segregation and PACE units for the seriously mentally ill, and crisis intervention teams to reduce uses of force.
But these innovations have touched only a small number of the incarcerated. The easy part has been designing and securing funding for these improvements. Actually implementing them has been tough and sometimes
impossible, in part because of the dilapidated state of the jails, but also as
a result of the disconnect between our electronic and DOC's paper-based
world, and the chaos of the larger jails like AMKC. The jails of Rikers simply
aren't up to the task of providing a safe and humane setting for either the
incarcerated or the people who work there.

Moving the jail staff and detainees into a few smaller, more modern jails
with proper information systems would create a boon to safety and productivity and allow reform to take hold. Such a move would also address
one of the most horrible aspects of Rikers—visitation. About 200,000 visitors come each year to see people held in the NYC jails, and the process
they endure to see their loved ones and friends is, much like incarceration
itself, arbitrary and humiliating. Visitors go through search and registration processes that change with every visit. Heightened stress and changing procedures can lead to misunderstandings, and minor disagreements
with security staff can result in being denied a visit. On the best day, visitors may travel from a central building to the visitor center and wait hours at
each spot, sometimes to be told that visits are not occurring. At one point in
2015, DOC proposed new visitation limits that included reductions on hugs
and allowances for children sitting on laps as a way to reduce contraband
getting into the jails. Fortunately, DOC backed off when the Board of Correction revealed data showing that fewer than 5 percent of seized weapons
came from the visit area and that the most consistent and serious source of
weapons was staff themselves.[20] Most systems as large as the NYC jails have
play areas for children, more efficient registration, and transparent rules and

appeals for visitation, but as one DOC official stated, "It's not a high priority right now."[21] A recent report by the advocacy group Jails Action Coalition detailed a gauntlet of sexual abuse, harassment, and profound humiliation that visitors to Rikers must endure.[22] One of the most disturbing findings of the report is that correctional officers use their authority and the desire of visitors to see their loved ones as leverage to sexually assault visitors under the guise of security searches. The report summarizes, "Women and men have reported being forced to strip down to their underwear, show COs their genitals, suffer through inappropriate touching of their breasts and genitals, and undergo cavity searches—even though these searches are directly in violation of DOC policy."

The ongoing abuse of visitors to Rikers reflects another truth of the NYC (and other) jail systems: reforms that reduce the rate of incarceration can occur while the plight of those who end up in jail is ignored. Having led the health service across two mayoral administrations, one a centrist Republican and the other a progressive Democrat, I have seen a remarkable consistency in how the incompetence of the correctional service was not only tolerated but also supported. At the core of these failings is a disconnect between policy makers in the mayor's office and other power structures and the pain that the jail system continues to deliver to those who pass through as detainees, visitors, and also staff. Reducing the rate of incarceration in NYC required much more than caring about the problem; it took a dedication to understanding the complex web of decisions starting with police and continuing to prosecutors, judges, and community treatment providers. In similar fashion, we need intelligent and accountable structural reform in Rikers and most of the nation's jails. This means transparency surrounding injuries and sexual assaults, as well as information systems that eliminate the ability of detainees to be "lost" or taken to remote spaces for physical or sexual abuse. This lack of transparency and accountability is much the same today as when I started in the jail system, and the lack of improvement in these contributors to health risks of jail stands in stark contrast to reforms outside the jails that have cut the rate of incarceration in half.

Closing Rikers will not eliminate the health risks of jail in NYC; some of these risks will always exist. But by closing Rikers and further reducing the jail population, we will stop hiding these health risks on a remote island. The ills of Rikers festered and devolved in large measure because they were completely removed from us. Community jails are more accessible to families, oversight, and government partners alike. Much of the abuse and neglect detailed in this book was facilitated by a practice of shuttling the person in question from one jail to another, creating confusion about where incidents occurred and who should investigate them. The abuse and humiliation experienced by visitors to Rikers Island are so established and accepted by city officials that they can only reflect a system functioning as designed, to repel all but the most intrepid loved ones and reduce contact and support between detainees and the outside world. Despite being a stone's throw from LaGuardia Airport, Rikers functions as a penal colony, where detainees are removed from their community, mostly because they are too poor to make bail, and where any perceived "problem" can be met with a dizzying array of jail transfers, opaque punishments, physical and sexual abuse, and further isolation from family members. Island penal colonies are designed for condemned people whom communities want to throw away and forget, and like Robben Island, Devil's Island, Saint Helena, and Alcatraz, the time has come for Rikers to close in favor of a smaller and more humane jail system. Closing Rikers will hinge on the ability of NYC and the state of New York to act in cooperation, as well as on the money to be made on real estate development. But NYC has very little affordable housing, and Rikers Island could provide sufficient space to create many thousands of affordable housing units while also developing the high-cost housing stock for the wealthy who control much of the city's agenda. Shining a light on the harms of jail in NYC has created a moment where closing Rikers has become a real possibility. In 2018, both NYC and the state of New York agree on this priority. We should jump at the opportunity.

Appendix

TABLE A.1. Cases, outcomes, and legal resolutions

Patient	Health outcome	Legal resolution
Bradley Ballard	Died of infection and dehydration after a week confined to a cell	$5.75 million settlement
Brianna	Reported being sexually assaulted in the women's jail	Pending class action lawsuit
Kalief Browder	Committed suicide after suffering physical abuse and solitary confinement over 3 years at Rikers; charges ultimately dropped	Pending lawsuit
Jason Echevarria	Died after ingestion of soap balls and denial of care	$3.8 million settlement; captain sentenced to 5 years in federal prison
Candie Hailey	Confined to solitary confinement for 27 of 29 months in Rikers	Pending lawsuit
Robert Hinton	Facial/neck injuries during use of force; killed in Brooklyn shooting in 2015	$450,000 settlement; captain and five officers fired
Jamal Lightfoot	Suffered multiple facial fractures after use of force initiated for making eye contact with senior security staff	$3.9 million settlement; security chief and six other security staff given sentences ranging from 4½ to 6½ years in prison
Maria	Reported being sexually assaulted in the women's jail	Pending class action lawsuit
Carlos Mercado	Died from diabetic ketoacidosis	$1.5 million settlement
Jerome Murdough	Died from heat stress when his cell overheated	$2.25 million settlement; one officer given probation
Angel Ramirez	Died from internal bleeding after use of force	$1.25 million settlement
Christopher Robinson	Died from internal bleeding after beating	$2 million settlement; two officers sentenced, one to 1 year in prison, the other to 2 years in prison
Ronald Spear	Died during use of force in the medical infirmary	$2.75 million settlement; two officers sentenced to 30 and 3 years in prison

TABLE A.2. Health outcomes for all jails to track and report publicly with standardized rates

Outcome	Variables
Injuries	All injuries, serious injuries, intentional injuries, those involving use of force, self-harm, those occurring in solitary and mental health settings, blow to head, location in jail
Deaths	Those considered jail attributable (any error in jail health or custody actions that contributes to death), withdrawal, homicide, accident, suicide, seizure, infection, chronic disease; deaths in first 72 hours of custody; overdose deaths in first 4 weeks after release from jail
Hospitalizations	Preventable (hospitalizations that result from lack of appropriate care in jail), delayed (lack of timely transfer), inappropriate returns (not clinically appropriate)
Serious mental illness, intellectual and developmental disability	Medication compliance, medication over objection, self-harm, suicide watch average length and number on watch, discharge planning and connection to care on reentry
Pharmacy	Access to medication when prescribed, lack of interruption of medications, access to community medications unless reasons clearly justified
Health encounters	Number of appointments scheduled and kept with reasons for not kept, tracking of sick call numbers
Health complaints/ grievances	Tracking of complaints that are substantiated (by outside review) and public reporting of every substantiated complaint in redacted form

Note: Standardized rates include, e.g., per 1,000 detainees, by gender and age category, or by LGBTQ status.

Notes

Introduction

1. While these personal experiences have formed my perspective, I've nonetheless selected the cases in each chapter based on the availability of sufficient public information to preclude me from passing along any protected or confidential information about any individual.
2. Estelle v. Gamble, 429 U.S. 97 (1976); see https://supreme.justia.com/cases /federal/us/429/97/case.html.
3. Venters H, Lainer-Vos J, Razvi A, Crawford J, Shaf'on Venable P, Drucker EM. Bringing health care advocacy to a public defender's office. *Am J Public Health*. 2008;98(11):1953–55.
4. Venters H, Razvi AM, Tobia MS, Drucker E. The case of Scott Ortiz: A clash between criminal justice and public health. *Harm Reduct J*. 2006;3:21. Available at https://harmreductionjournal.biomedcentral.com/articles/10.1186 /1477-7517-3-21.
5. Venters HD, US House of Representatives, House Judiciary Committee's Subcommittee on Immigration, Citizenship, Refugees, Border Security, and International Law. Hearing on Problems with Immigration Detainee Medical Care, June 4, 2008. Available at www.aila.org/File/Related /08060432Venters.pdf.
6. Bernstein N. Another jail death, and mounting questions. *New York Times*. Jan. 27, 2009. www.nytimes.com/2009/01/28/us/28detain.html?_r=0.
7. Venters H, Dasch-Goldberg D, Rasmussen A, Keller AS. Into the abyss: Mortality and morbidity among detained immigrants. *Human Rights Quarterly*. 2009;31(2):474–95.
8. Venters et al., Into the abyss.
9. Siegel B. *A Death in White Bear Lake: The True Chronicle of An All-American Town*. New York: Ballantine Books; 2000.
10. State v. Loss, 204 N.W.2d 404 (1973); see http://law.justia.com/cases /minnesota/supreme-court/1973/43421-1.html.
11. Minton TD. *Jail Inmates at Midyear 2010—Statistical Tables*. Washington, DC: US Department of Justice; 2011. https://www.bjs.gov/content/pub/pdf /jim10st.pdf. Austin J, Naro-Ware W, Ocker R, Harris R, Allen R. *Evaluation of the Current and Future Los Angeles County Jail Population*. Denver, CO: JFA Institute; 2012. http://www.jfa-associates.com/publications/ppsm/Los %20Angeles%20Jail%20Projections.pdf. Olson DE, Tahier S. *Population Dynamics and the Characteristics of Inmates in the Cook County Jail*. Chicago: Cook

County Sheriff's Reentry Council; 2012. https://ecommons.luc.edu/cgi /viewcontent.cgi?article=1003&context=criminaljustice_facpubs.

Chapter 1. Dying in Jail

1. Final Report of the New York State Commission of Correction; In the Matter of the Death of Carlos Mercado, an inmate of the Anna M. Kross Center. December 16, 2014 (Redacted). Brown S. Family of diabetic Rikers Island inmate who died to receive $1.5M settlement. *New York Daily News*. Nov. 30, 2015.
2. Sheldon S. The scary story of diabetic ketoacidosis. *Loop*. Feb. 18, 2013. www.loop-blog.com/the-scary-experience-of-diabetic-ketoacidosis/.
3. Small E. Rikers Jail medical provider let inmate die from diabetic coma, suit says. *DNAinfo*. Aug. 21, 2014.
4. Brittain J, Axelrod G, Venters H. Deaths in New York City jails: 2001–2009. *Am J Public Health*. 2013;103:4.
5. What were your worst experiences with alcohol withdrawal? Reddit alcoholism. Available at www.reddit.com/r/alcoholism/comments/3b8eza/what _were_your_worst_experiences_with_alcohol/.
6. Pearson J. In deadly NYC jail beatings, no criminal charges. Associated Press. Aug. 21, 2014. http://www.oneidadispatch.com/general-news/20140820 /guards-not-punished-for-beating-killing-inmates.
7. Lim S, Seligson AL, Parvez FM, Luther CW, Mavinkurve MP, Binswanger IA, Kerker BD. Risks of drug-related death, suicide, and homicide during the immediate post-release period among people released from New York City jails, 2001–2005. *Am J Epidemiol*. 2012;175(6):519–26.
8. *Neither Justice nor Treatment: Drug Courts in the United States*. Physicians for Human Rights. June 2017. http://physiciansforhumanrights.org/assets /misc/phr_drugcourts_report_singlepages.pdf.
9. Gisev N, Larney S, Kimber J, Burns L, Weatherburn D, Gibson A, Dobbins T, Mattick R, Butler T, Degenhardt L. Determining the impact of opioid substitution therapy upon mortality and recidivism among prisoners: A 22 year data linkage study. Trends & issues in crime and criminal justice no. 498. June 3, 2015. https://aic.gov.au/publications/tandi/tandi498.
10. Sommerfeldt C. Sheriff David Clarke, one of Donald Trump's cabinet considerations, hurled threats over suspicious jail deaths. *New York Daily News*. Dec. 2, 2016. www.nydailynews.com/news/politics/potential-trump-pick -david-clarke-hurled-threats-jail-deaths-article-1.2895326.
11. Yeung B. Taser's delirium defense: How lawyers used junk science to explain away stun-gun deaths. *Mother Jones*. Mar./Apr. 2009. www.motherjones.com /politics/2009/02/tasers-delirium-defense.
12. Lithwick D. Dying of excitement. *Slate*. June 11, 2014. http://www.slate.com

/articles/news_and_politics/jurisprudence/2015/06/excited_delirium _deaths_in_police_custody_diagnosis_or_cover_up.html.

13. Cartwright S. Report on the diseases and peculiarities of the Negro race. *New Orleans Medical and Surgical Journal.* May 1851.

14. Granski M, Keller A, Venters H. Death rates among detained immigrants in the United States. *Int J Environ Res Public Health.* 2015;12(11):14414–19. https:// www.ncbi.nlm.nih.gov/pmc/articles/PMC4661656/.

15. *The Enhanced Pre-arraignment Screening Unit: Improving Health Services, Medical Triage, and Diversion Opportunities in Manhattan Central Booking.* Vera Institute of Justice. Sept. 2017. https://www.vera.org/publications/the-enhanced-pre -arraignment-screening-unit.

Chapter 2. Injury and Violence

1. Parkes J. A review of the literature on positional asphyxia as a possible cause of sudden death during restraint. *Br J Forens Pract.* 2002;4(1):24–30.

2. Chan TC, Vilke GM, Neuman T, Clausen JL. Restraint position and positional asphyxia. *Ann Emerg Med.* 1997;30(5):578–86. doi:10.1016/S0196-0644(97) 70072-6. Stratton JS, Rogers C, Green K. Sudden death in individuals in hobble restraints during paramedic transport. *Ann Emerg Med.* 1995;25(5): 710–12.

3. Medical examiner rules Eric Garner's death a homicide, says he was killed by chokehold. *NBC 4 New York.* Aug. 1, 2014. www.nbcnewyork.com/news/local /Eric-Garner-Chokehold-Police-Custody-Cause-of-Death-Staten-Island -Medical-Examiner-269396151.html.

4. Judge recommends firing officers in Rikers beating case. *New York Times.* Sept. 29, 2014. www.nytimes.com/interactive/2014/09/30/nyregion/judges -recommendation-on-rikers-case.html. Weiser B. New York to settle suit over Rikers inmate whom guards attacked. *New York Times.* Sept. 2, 2015. www.nytimes.com/2015/09/03/nyregion/new-york-to-settle-suit-over -rikers-inmate-whom-guards-attacked.html.

5. Schwirtz M. Former Rikers inmate who received settlement is fatally shot in Brooklyn. *New York Times.* Nov. 27, 2015. www.nytimes.com/2015/11/28 /nyregion/former-rikers-inmate-who-received-settlement-is-fatally-shot-in -brooklyn.html.

6. Ludwig A, Parsons, A, Cohen, L, Venters H. Injury surveillance in the NYC jail system. *Am J Public Health.* 2012;102(6):1108–11.

7. Glowa-Kollisch S, Andrade K, Stazesky R, Teixeira P, Kaba F, MacDonald R, Rosner Z, Selling D, Parsons A, Venters H. Data-driven human rights: Using the electronic health record to promote human rights in jail. *Health and Human Rights.* 2014;16(1):157–65.

8. Pearson J. Official: More NYC inmates splashing health staff. Associated Press. Jan. 16, 2004. www.correctionsone.com/correctional-healthcare/articles /6743739-Official-More-NYC-inmates-splashing-health-staff/.

9. Winerip M, Schwirtz M. Rikers: Where mental illness meets brutality in jail. *New York Times.* July 14, 2014. www.nytimes.com/2014/07/14/nyregion /rikers-study-finds-prisoners-injured-by-employees.html.

10. Winerip M, Schwirtz M, Weiser B. Report found distorted data on jail fights at Rikers Island. *New York Times.* Sept. 21, 2014. www.nytimes.com/2014/09 /22/nyregion/report-twisted-data-on-fights-in-a-rikers-jail.html.

11. Moynihanjan C. Two officers sentenced in Rikers Island assault case. *New York Times.* Jan. 17, 2012. www.nytimes.com/2012/01/18/nyregion/rikers-island -officers-sentenced-in-assault-case.html.

12. Watson AC, Fulambarker AJ. The crisis intervention team model of police response to mental health crises: A primer for mental health practitioners. *Best Pract Ment Health.* 2012;8(2):71.

13. Steiner A. Minnesota's Barbara Schneider Foundation teaches crisis interven-tion strategies to Rikers Island team. *MinnPost.* July 17, 2015. www.minnpost .com/mental-health-addiction/2015/07/minnesota-s-barbara-schneider -foundation-teaches-crisis-intervention.

Chapter 3. Solitary Confinement

1. Schwirtz M. U.S. accuses Rikers officer of ignoring dying plea. *New York Times.* Mar. 24, 2014. www.nytimes.com/2014/03/25/nyregion/correction-officer -charged-with-indifference-in-death-of-rikers-island-inmate.html?_r=0.

2. Biggs BS. Solitary confinement: A brief history. *Mother Jones.* Mar. 2, 2009. www.motherjones.com/politics/2009/03/solitary-confinement-brief -natural-history.

3. Dickens C. *American Notes for Circulation.* London: Chapman & Hall; 1842.

4. Medley, Petitioner, 134 U.S. 160, 161 (1890).

5. Peters J. How a 1983 murder created America's terrible supermax-prison culture. *Slate.* Oct. 23, 2013. www.slate.com/blogs/crime/2013/10/23/marion _prison_lockdown_thomas_silverstein_how_a_1983_murder_created _america.html.

6. Kuppers T. *Expert Report of Terry A. Kupers, MD, MSP.* East Mississippi Correc-tional Facility. June 14, 2015. Haney C. Mental health issues in long-term solitary and "supermax" confinement. *Crime and Delinquency.* 2003;49(1).

7. Kaba F, Lewsi A, Glowa-Kollisch S, Hadler J, Lee D, Alper H, Selling D, MacDonald R, Solimo A, Parsons A, Venters H. Solitary confinement and risk of self-harm among jail inmates. *Amer J Public Health.* 2014;104(3):442–47.

8. NYC Department of Correction closes mental health assessment unit for

infracted inmates. NYC DOC press release. Jan. 6, 2014. www.nyc.gov/html /doc/downloads/pdf/press-releases/jan6-2014.pdf.

9. US Department of Justice complaint re abuse of adolescents. Aug. 4, 2014. "Shortly after our second site visit in April 2013, DOC made the long overdue decision to stop placing infracted mentally ill adolescents in MHAUII. MHAUII was an inappropriate setting for any inmate suffering from mental illness, particularly adolescents. The conditions were deplorable, the physical facilities were in disrepair, and adolescents were not separated by sight and sound from adult offenders as required by correctional standards. It was evident that the adolescents were at risk of psychologically decompensating due to the corrosive environment. Several of the most egregious use of force incidents occurred at MHAUII. At the end of 2013, DOC finally closed the entire unit" (47).

10. Pearson J. Inmates in solitary more likely to hurt themselves. Associated Press. Feb. 12, 2014. www.ksl.com/?sid=28695131. Northridge M, Holtzman D. Paper and Reviewer of the Year award winners. *Am J Public Health*. 2014;104(11): e8–e11. http://ajph.aphapublications.org/doi/abs/10.2105/AJPH.2014 .302255.

11. Western District, Pelican Bay class action; case no. 4:09 CV 05796 CW. Expert testimony of Dr. Craig Haney, reference 29. Southern District, Nunez class action; case no. 14 CV 8672, original filing, 29. Submission to the United Nations Universal Periodic Review of United States of America, 2nd cycle, Human Rights Council, April–May 2015. Center for Constitutional Rights, Legal Services for Prisoners with Children, California Prison Focus. Ref. 5. New York Advisory Committee to the U.S. Commission on Civil Rights. The Solitary Confinement of Youth in New York. Dec. 14. Ref. 258.

12. Morris R. Exploring the effect of exposure to short-term solitary confinement among violent prison inmates. *J Quant Crim*. 2016;32(1):1–22.

13. Davis v. Ayala, 576 U.S. ___ (2015), Concurrence, Anthony M. Kennedy.

Chapter 4. Serious Mental Illness in Jail

1. Pearson J. Inmate died after 7 days in Rikers Island cell: AP. *NBC 4 New York*. May 22, 2014. https://www.nbcnewyork.com/news/local/AP-Bradley-Ballard -Died-Rikers-Cell-NYC-Corrections-260220681.html.

2. http://documentslide.com/documents/scoc-death-reports-on-polo -gionnotta-and-moore.html

3. Hutchinson B. Blau R. Rikers Island inmate who hanged himself on New Year's Day should have been on suicide watch. *New York Daily News*. Jan. 2, 2015. www.nydailynews.com/new-york/nyc-crime/sex-offender-rikers-island -hangs-prison-cell-article-1.2064056.

4. Leid C. Man dies in Rikers Island cell, family says he was denied anti-seizure medication. *ABC 7 New York*. Nov. 1, 2016. http://abc7ny.com/news /exclusive-man-dies-in-rikers-island-cell-family-says-he-was-denied -medication/1584631/.

5. Ford E. *Sometimes Amazing Things Happen: Heartbreak and Hope on the Bellevue Hospital Psychiatric Prison Ward*. New York: Simon & Schuster; 2017.

6. *No Room at the Inn: Trends and Consequences of Closing Public Psychiatric Hospitals*. Treatment Advocacy Center; July 2012. http://www.treatmentadvocacycenter .org/storage/documents/no_room_at_the_inn-2012.pdf.

7. Cost of inmate in NYC almost as much as Ivy League tuition. Associated Press. Sept. 30, 2013. www.nydailynews.com/new-york/cost-inmate-nyc-ivy -league-tuition-article-1.1471630.

8. Substance Abuse and Mental Health Services Administration. *Housing Options for Adults with Mental and Substance Use Disorders Involved with the Criminal Justice System*. Evidence-Based Practices and Criminal Justice Series. Rockville, MD: Substance Abuse and Mental Health Services Administration; 2016. https:// www.prainc.com/wp-content/uploads/2016/10/housing072616.pdf.

9. *Frequent Users Service Enhancement 'FUSE' Initiative*. New York City FUSE II Evaluation Report. Center for Housing Solutions and Columbia Mailman School of Public Health. Mar. 2014. https://shnny.org/uploads/CSH-FUSE -Evaluation.pdf.

10. Weiser B. City to pay $5.75 million over death of mentally ill inmate at Rikers Island. *New York Times*. Sept. 27, 2016. https://www.nytimes.com/2016/09/28 /nyregion/rikers-island-lawsuit-bradley-ballard.html.

Chapter 5. Human Rights and Correctional Health

1. Deutsch K. Bronx woman arrested for stabbing a 3-month-old girl during a wild argument with the baby's mother. *New York Daily News*. Feb. 22, 2012. www.nydailynews.com/new-york/bronx/bronx-woman-arrested-stabbing -3-year-old-girl-wild-argument-girl-mother-article-1.1026951.

2. Pearson J. After years in solitary, a woman struggles to carry on. Associated Press. Feb. 17, 2016. www.apnews.com/44c62b6377c34851895032caa6b3d592.

3. Physicians for Human Rights. *Dual Loyalty and Human Rights in Health Professional Practice: Proposed Guidelines and Institutional Mechanisms*. March 2003. Available at https://s3.amazonaws.com/PHR_Reports/dualloyalties-2002 -report.pdf. Pont J, Stover H, Wolf H. Dual loyalty in prison health care. *Am J Public Health*. 2012;102(3):475–80.

4. Allen M. Colorado prison guards joke while mentally ill inmate dies. *Denver Post*. June 20, 2014. https://www.denverpost.com/2014/06/19/family-of -mentally-ill-inmate-says-guards-laughed-and-joked-as-he-died/.

5. St. John P. Naked, filthy and strapped to a chair for 46 hours: A mentally ill inmate's last days. *LA Times.* Aug. 24, 2017. www.latimes.com/local/california /la-me-jails-mentally-ill-20170824-story.html.

6. Winerip M, Schwirtz M. An inmate dies, and no one is punished. *New York Times.* Dec. 13, 2015. www.nytimes.com/2015/12/14/nyregion/clinton -correctional-facility-inmate-brutality.html.

7. MacDonald R, Parsons A, Venters H. The triple aims of correctional health: Patient safety, population health and human rights. *J Health Care Poor Underserved.* 2013;24(3):1226–34.

8. Weiser B. Rikers officer pleads guilty to helping cover up fatal '12 beating of inmate. *New York Times.* Sept. 20, 2016. www.nytimes.com/2016/09/21 /nyregion/rikers-island-beating-ronald-spear.html?_r=0.

9. Mualimm-ak FO. Solitary confinement's invisible scars. *Guardian.* Oct. 30, 2013. www.theguardian.com/commentisfree/2013/oct/30/solitary -confinement-invisible-scars.

10. NYC Board of Correction Meeting. Dec. 15, 2015. Available at www.youtube .com/watch?v=bREInoRx3fY.

11. Glowa-Kollisch S, Graves J, Dickey N, MacDonald R, Rosner Z, Waters A, Venters H. Data-driven human rights: Using dual loyalty trainings to promote the care of vulnerable patients in jail. *Health Hum Rights.* 2015;17(1):E124-35.

12. Glowa-Kollisch et al., Data-driven human rights, 126.

13. Glowa-Kollisch et al., Data-driven human rights, 131.

14. Report of US Department of Justice, US Attorney for the Southern District of New York regarding NYC Jail System. Aug. 4, 2014. https://www.justice .gov/sites/default/files/usao-sdny/legacy/2015/03/25/SDNY%20Rikers %20Report.pdf.

15. Glowa-Kollisch S, Andrade K, Stazesky R, Teixeira P, Kaba F, MacDonald R, Rosner Z, Selling D, Parsons A, Venters H. Data-driven human rights: Using the electronic health record to promote human rights in jail. *Health Hum Rights.* 2014;16(1):157–65.

16. Principles of Medical Ethics. UN Doc No. A/RES/37/194. Dec. 18, 1982. Principle 2. Available at www.un.org/documents/ga/res/37/a37r194.htm.

Chapter 6. Race

1. Schiraldi V. How to reduce crime: Stop charging children as adults. *New York Times.* Feb. 26, 2016. www.nytimes.com/2016/02/26/opinion/how-to-reduce -crime-stop-charging-children-as-adults.html.

2. Rayman G. Rikers fight club: The knockout punch. *Village Voice.* Apr. 15, 2009.

3. CRIPA investigation of the New York City Department of Correction jails on Rikers Island. US Department of Justice. Aug. 4, 2014. www.justice.gov

/sites/default/files/usao-sdny/legacy/2015/03/25/SDNY%20Rikers%20
Report.pdf.
4. Gonnerman J. Before the law: A boy was accused of taking a backpack.
The courts took the next three years of his life. *New Yorker*. Oct. 6, 2014.
www.newyorker.com/magazine/2014/10/06/before-the-law.
5. Moynihanjan C. Two officers sentenced in Rikers Island assault case. *New York
Times*. Jan. 17, 2012. www.nytimes.com/2012/01/18/nyregion/rikers-island
-officers-sentenced-in-assault-case.html?mtrref=www.google.com&gwh
=C013EDF1B5463BD5CB663AD46EA25BDC&gwt=pay.
6. Winerip M, Schwirtz M, Weiser B. Report found distorted data on jail fights
at Rikers Island. *New York Times*. Sept. 21, 2014. www.nytimes.com/2014/09/22
/nyregion/report-twisted-data-on-fights-in-a-rikers-jail.html.
7. Kaba F, Solimo A, Graves J, Glowa-Kollisch S, Vise A, MacDonald R, Waters A,
Rosner Z, Dickey N, Angell S, Venters H. Disparities in mental health referral
and diagnosis in the NYC jail mental health service. *Am J Public Health*. 2015;
105(9):1911–16.
8. Manseau M, Case B. Racial-ethnic disparities in outpatient mental health
visits to U.S. physicians, 1993–2008. *Psychiatr Serv*. 2014;65(1):59–67.
9. Public Broadcasting Corporation: Africans in America. Diseases and peculiarities of the Negro race. https://www.pbs.org/wgbh/aia/part4/4h3106t.html.
10. *Barriers to Recreation*. NYC Board of Correction. July 2014. https://www
.prisonpolicy.org/scans/CPSU_Rec_Report.pdf.
11. Graves J, Steele J, Kaba F, Ramdath C, Rosner Z, MacDonald R, Dickey N,
Venters H. Traumatic brain injury and structural violence among adolescent
males in the NYC jail system. *J Health Care Poor Underserved*. 2015;26(2):345–57.
12. Kaba F, Diamond P, Haque A, MacDonald R, Venters H. Traumatic brain
injury among newly admitted adolescents in the New York City jail system.
J Adolesc Health. 2014;54(5):615–17.
13. Gonnerman J. Kalief Browder, 1993–2015. *New Yorker*. June 7, 2015.
www.newyorker.com/news/news-desk/kalief-browder-1993-2015.
14. Siegler A, Rosner Z, MacDonald R, Ford E, Venters H. Head trauma in jail
and implications for chronic traumatic encephalopathy in the United States:
Case report and results of injury surveillance in NYC jails. *J Health Care Poor
Underserved*. 2017;28(3):1042–49. doi:10.1353/hpu.2017.0095.
15. Hetey RC, Eberhardt J. Racial disparities in incarceration increase acceptance
of punitive policies. *Psychol Sci*. 2014;25(10):1949–54. Ghandnoosh N. *Race
and Punishment: Racial Perceptions of Crime and Support for Punitive Policies*.
Washington, DC: The Sentencing Project; 2014. http://sentencingproject.org
/doc/publications/rd_Race_and_Punishment.pdf.

16. Office of the Surgeon General, Center for Mental Health Services, National Institute of Mental Health. Mental health: Culture, race and ethnicity. A supplement to Mental health: A report of the surgeon general. Rockville, MD: Substance Abuse and Mental Health Services Administration; 2001.

17. Baillargeon J, Penn J, Thomas C, Temple J, Baillargeon G, Murray O. Psychiatric disorders and suicide in the nation's largest state prison system. *J Am Acad Psychiatry Law*. 2009;37(2):188–93. Karnik NS, Soller M, Redlich A, Silverman MA, Kraemer HC, Haapanen R, Steiner H. Prevalence differences of psychiatric disorders among youth after nine months or more of incarceration by race/ethnicity and age. *J Health Care Poor Underserved*. 2010;21(1):237–50. Karnik NS, Jones P, Campanero A, Haapanen R, Steiner H. Ethnic variation of self-reported psychopathology among incarcerated youth. *Community Ment Health J*. 2006;42(5):477–86.

18. Criminologist challenges the effectiveness of solitary confinement. UT Dallas News Center. Mar. 31, 2015. www.utdallas.edu/news/2015/3/31-31472 _Criminologist-Challenges-the-Effectiveness-of-Soli_story-wide.html?WT .mc_id=NewsHomePage.

19. SPNS Initiative: Culturally appropriate interventions of outreach, access and retention among Latino(a) populations, 2013–2018. H97HA27431-01-00 for Special Projects of National Significance to New York, City of (the), Long Island City, New York, is provided by the Health Resources and Services Administration. 2014. Available at http://hab.hrsa.gov/abouthab/special /latino.html#3.

20. Nobles WP. ACLU sues Orleans Public Defenders office over refusal of cases. *NOLA.com | Times-Picayune*. Jan. 15, 2016. www.nola.com/crime/index.ssf /2016/01/aclu_sues_orleans_public_defen.html.

Chapter 7. Sexual Assault in Rikers

1. Maria and Brianna are pseudonyms for Jane Doe 1 and Jane Doe 2, who filed suit on behalf of themselves and similarly situated women v. The City of New York and Benny Santiago. US District Court, Southern District of New York. 15 CV 03849 (AKH). Unless otherwise specified, all information relating to these cases is drawn from this source.

2. Beck A, Berezofsky M. Sexual victimization in prisons and jails reported by inmates, 2011–12. Bureau of Justice Statistics, US Department of Justice. May 2013. NCJ 241399.

3. *Correctional Health Quarterly Reports on Sexual Assault*. Released by N.Y. Public Advocate Leticia James. Available at http://pubadvocate.nyc.gov/sites /advocate.nyc.gov/files/james_declaration_exhibits.pdf.

4. CRIPA investigation of the New York City Department of Correction jails on Rikers Island, letter to Mayor DeBlasio from US Attorney Preet Bharara, p. 10, n. 14.

5. Case history of Rodney Hulin. *No Escape: Male Rape in U.S. Prisons Human Rights Watch Report.* April 2001. www.hrw.org/legacy/reports/2001/prison/rodney _hulin.html.

6. Eligon J. A repeat escapee receives a lengthy sentence. *New York Times.* July 21, 2011. www.nytimes.com/2011/07/22/nyregion/repeat-escapee-ronald -tackman-gets-long-prison-sentence.html.

7. Former inmate sneaks back into jail at Rikers Island and impersonates Department of Corrections employee. *PIX11 New York.* Mar. 1, 2013. http://pix11.com /2013/03/01/pix-exclusive-fake-rikers-corrections-officer-arrested/.

8. Ng P. Dept. of Investigation probe finds poor security at Rikers Island. *PIX11 New York.* Nov. 6, 2014. http://pix11.com/2014/11/06/probe-finds-poor -security-at-rikers-island/.

9. Rayman G. Rikers con job. *Village Voice.* Aug. 8, 2012. https://www.villagevoice .com/2012/08/08/rikers-con-job/.

10. Hoffer J. Investigators' exclusive: Rikers inmate alleges correction officer sex abuse. *ABC 7 New York.* June 30, 2016. http://abc7ny.com/news/investigators -exclusive-rikers-inmate-alleges-guard-sex-abuse/1405543/.

11. The criminal justice system: Statistics. RAINN. www.rainn.org/statistics /criminal-justice-system.

12. NYC Board of Correction public meeting. Nov. 15, 2016. Available at www .youtube.com/watch?v=QqebeB7rI-U&feature=youtu.be, at the 32-minute mark.

13. Exhibits for declaration of NYC Public Advocate Leticia James. Case 1:15-cv-03848-AKH. Filed Oct. 9, 2015. Available at http://advocate.nyc.gov/sites /advocate.nyc.gov/files/james_declaration_exhibits.pdf.

14. Rodriguez C. Reports of sexual abuse against Rikers inmates rise. *WNYC News.* May 26, 2016. www.wnyc.org/story/reports-sexual-abuse-rikers-concern -medical-staff/.

15. Available at www.thenation.com/wp-content/uploads/2015/04/rick_perry _letter.pdf.

16. Available at https://www.scribd.com/document/236254571/Pence-Letter -To-Eric-Holder.

17. Tcholakian D. City jails will comply with federal rape guidelines that were set in 2003. *DNAinfo.* Nov. 15, 2016. www.dnainfo.com/new-york/20161115/civic -center/new-york-city-board-department-correction-sexual-assauly-jail.

18. Jaffer M, Ayad J, Tungol JG, MacDonald R, Dickey N, Venters H. Improving

transgender healthcare in the New York City correctional system. *LGBT Health*. 2016 Apr;3(2):116–21.

Chapter 8. Correctional Health

1. Murphy B. Nassau sheriff stands by jail health care provider Armor. *Newsday*. Sept. 10, 2016. www.newsday.com/long-island/nassau/nassau-sheriff-stands -by-jail-health-care-provider-armor-1.12296093. Officials: Nassau County Jail inmate dies; 6th this year. *NEWS12 Long Island*. Updated Sept. 7, 2016. https:// www.brewingtonlaw.com/sites/default/files/pressclips2016/Officials-Nassau -County-Jail-inmate-dies-6th-this-year-News-12-Long-Island.pdf. Rates were compared using the first six months of 2016, with 1,100 inmates and six deaths; rate was approximately 11 per 1,000 inmates per year. In NYC, the rate has been 1–2 per 1,000 inmates per year for about five years, and the national average is about 2–3 per 1,000.

2. Press E. Madness: In Florida prisons, mentally ill inmates have been tortured, driven to suicide, and killed by guards. *New Yorker*. May 2, 2016. www .newyorker.com/magazine/2016/05/02/the-torturing-of-mentally-ill -prisoners.

Chapter 9. Transparency and Governance

1. www1.nyc.gov/assets/boc/downloads/pdf/BOCMinutes%20(3.12.12).pdf
2. Glowa-Kollisch S, Kaba F, Waters A, Leung YJ, Ford E, Venters H. From punishment to treatment: The "Clinical Alternative to Punitive Segregation" (CAPS) program in New York City jails. *Int J Environ Res Public Health*. 2016;13(2):182.
3. Lee B, Gilligan J, Report to the NYC BOC. Sept. 5, 2013. http://nycjac.org /report-to-the-nyc-boc-by-drs-james-gilligan-and-bandy-lee/.
4. Brown SR, Blau R. Correction officers "relish confrontation" and keep using violent force against Rikers inmates, report reveals. *New York Daily News*. Oct. 11, 2017. www.nydailynews.com/new-york/manhattan/rikers-staff -relish-conflict-violence-inmates-report-article-1.3554355.
5. Rayman G. Rikers con job. *Village Voice*. Aug. 8, 2012. https://www.villagevoice .com/2012/08/08/rikers-con-job/.
6. Calder R. Rikers guards to get lessons on how to talk nicely to inmates. *New York Post*. Nov. 4, 2016. http://nypost.com/2016/11/04/rikers-guards-to-get -lessons-on-how-to-talk-nicely-to-inmates/.
7. Sedlak AJ, McPherson KS. Conditions of confinement: Findings from the survey of youth in residential placement. *Juvenile Justice Bulletin*. May 2010. www.ncjrs.gov/pdffiles1/ojjdp/227729.pdf.

8. Istanbul Protocol, Office of the High Commissioner for Human Rights, United Nations, 1991 and 2004. https://www.scribd.com/document/37338684 /Istanbul-Protocol.

9. *Sex Workers at Risk: Condoms as Evidence of Prostitution in Four US Cities.* Human Rights Watch. July 19, 2012. https://www.hrw.org/report/2012/07/19/sex -workers-risk/condoms-evidence-prostitution-four-us-cities.

10. Parvez F, Katyal M, Alper H, Leibowitz R, Venters H. Female sex workers incarcerated in New York City jails: Prevalence of sexually transmitted infections and associated risk behaviors. *Sex Transm Infect.* 2013;89(4): 280–84.

11. Jorgensen J. Council passes Rikers Island health reporting bill. *Observer.* May 27, 2015. http://observer.com/2015/05/council-passes-rikers-island -health-reporting-bill/.

12. Liu S, Watcha D, Holodniy M, Goldhaber-Fiebert JD. Sofosbuvir-based treatment regimens for chronic, genotype 1 hepatitis C virus infection in U.S. incarcerated populations: A cost-effectiveness analysis. *Ann Intern Med.* 2014;161(8):546–53.

Conclusion

1. Goodman JD. De Blasio says idea of closing Rikers jail complex is unrealistic. *New York Times.* Feb. 16, 2016. www.nytimes.com/2016/02/17/nyregion/ de-blasio-says-idea-of-closing-rikers-jail-complex-is-unrealistic.html?_r=0.

2. Fermino J. First Lady Chirlane McCray says she thinks closing Rikers Island is a "great idea"—a day after Mayor de Blasio said he'd rather fix the jail. *New York Daily News.* Feb. 17, 2016. www.nydailynews.com/new-york/queens/nyc -lady-breaks-husband-favors-closing-rikers-article-1.2535327.

3. Mark M. New York City is set to close the first of its notorious Rikers Island jails this summer. *Business Insider.* Jan. 2, 2018. www.businessinsider.com /first-rikers-jail-to-close-this-summer-2018-1.

4. Schwirtz M, Winerip M. Close Rikers Island? It Will Take Years, Billions and Political Capital. *New York Times.* Mar. 2, 2016. www.nytimes.com/2016/03/03 /nyregion/closing-rikers-island-despite-rhetoric-intractable-obstacles -remain.html?_r=0.

5. LICH's clumsy closing: A fruitless fight in Brooklyn cost SUNY about $100 million. Editorial. *Crain's New York Business.* June 20, 2014. www.crainsnewyork .com/article/20140620/OPINION/140629990/lichs-clumsy-closing.

6. Here are city documents on "effort" to close Rikers that de Blasio denies. *DNAinfo.* Apr. 14, 2016. www.dnainfo.com/new-york/20160414/college-point /here-are-city-documents-on-effort-close-rikers-that-de-blasio-denies.

7. O'Brien RD. Portrait of the frequently jailed: Have big problems, do minor

crimes. *Wall Street Journal*. Sept. 17, 2015. www.wsj.com/articles/portrait-of
-the-frequently-jailed-have-big-problems-do-minor-crimes-1442520060.

8. King DH. Bronx program serves as inspiration for Mark-Viverito's city-wide
   bail fund proposal. *Gotham Gazette*. Feb. 20, 2015. www.gothamgazette.com
   /index.php/government/5588-bronx-program-serves-as-inspiration-for
   -mark-viveritos-city-wide-bail-fund-proposal.

9. Mayor de Blasio and Chief Judge Lippman announce Justice Reboot, an
   initiative to modernize the criminal justice system. City of New York website.
   www1.nyc.gov/office-of-the-mayor/news/235-15/mayor-de-blasio-chief
   -judge-lippman-justice-reboot-initiative-modernize-the.

10. Parry B. Reforms created after Kalief Browder's death have failed: Lancman.
    TimesLedger. Nov. 4, 2016. www.timesledger.com/stories/2016/45
    /browderlancman_2016_11_04_q.html.

11. Bail fail: Why the U.S. should end the practice of using money for bail. Justice
    Policy Institute. Sept. 2012. www.justicepolicy.org/uploads/justicepolicy
    /documents/bailfail_executive_summary.pdf.

12. Marimow AE. When it comes to pretrial release, few other jurisdictions do it
    D.C.'s way. *Washington Post*. July 4, 2016. www.washingtonpost.com/local
    /public-safety/when-it-comes-to-pretrial-release-few-other-jurisdictions-do
    -it-dcs-way/2016/07/04/8eb52134-e7d3-11e5-b0fd-073d5930a7b7_story.html.

13. www.ibo.nyc.ny.us/iboreports/pretrialdetainneltrsept2011.pdf

14. Fractenberg B, Small E. City moving 16-, 17-year-olds off Rikers to new Bronx
    facility, mayor says. *DNAinfo*. July 21, 2016. www.dnainfo.com/new-york
    /20160721/melrose/city-moving-16-17-year-olds-off-rikers-new-bronx
    -facility-mayor-says.

15. Calder R, Gonen Y. Rikers trains guards in prohibited eye gouges, elbow
    strikes. *New York Post*. Aug. 22, 2016. http://nypost.com/2016/08/22/rikers
    -trains-guards-in-prohibited-eye-gouges-elbow-strikes/.

16. Husamudeen E. For immediate release: COBA president Elias Husamudeen
    regarding the DOC's elimination of punitive segregation for 18–21 year old
    inmates. Correctional Officers' Benevolent Association. www.cobanyc.org
    /news/immediate-release-coba-president-elias-husamudeen-regarding
    -doc%E2%80%99s-elimination-punitive.

17. US Department of Justice. *CRIPA Investigation of the New York City Department
    of Correction Jails on Rikers Island*. Aug. 4, 2014. www.justice.gov/sites/default
    /files/usao-sdny/legacy/2015/03/25/SDNY%20Rikers%20Report.pdf.

18. Blau R. Violence rate in city jails spike despite record spending and drop
    in detainees, analysis shows. *New York Daily News*. Nov. 28, 2016. www
    .nydailynews.com/new-york/nyc-crime/violence-city-jails-spike-drop
    -detainees-analysis-article-1.2890111.

19. Brown SR, Blau R. Rikers Island correction bosses routinely "purge" unfavorable violence stats to create illusion of reform, review shows. *New York Daily News*. Aug. 28, 2016. www.nydailynews.com/new-york/exclusive-rikers-island-bosses-cover-violence-stats-article-1.2768232.

20. Law V. No touching: Relatives of Rikers inmates protest proposed visitation rules. Gothamist. Sept. 9, 2015. http://gothamist.com/2015/09/09/rikers_physical_contact.php.

21. Blakinger K, Blau R. Visitors struggle with hours-long waits, multiple checkpoints on Rikers Island. *New York Daily News*. Jan. 18, 2016. www.nydailynews.com/new-york/visitors-struggle-hours-long-waits-rikers-island-article-1.2500063.

22. *"It makes me want to cry": Visiting Rikers Island*. NYC Jails Action Coalition. Jan. 2018. http://nycjac.org/wp-content/uploads/2018/01/VISITING-RIKERS-ISLAND-JAILS-ACTION-COALITION-1.9.18.pdf.

Index